Face The Pain

The Challenge of Facial Pain

Wesley E. Shankland, II, D.D.S., M.S., Ph.D.

http://www.drshankland.com

Revised 2001

~ AOmega Publishing Co. ~
Columbus, Ohio

Face The Pain

The Challenge of Facial Pain

Wesley E. Shankland, II, D.D.S., M.S. Ph.D.

AOmega Publishing Co.
Columbus, Ohio 43231
614-794-0033

The material in *Face The Pain* is presented for informational purposes only and it is not meant to be, and should not be relied upon, for recommendations regarding diagnosis and treatment for any individual case. It is not meant to be a substitute for proper medical care by your doctor. You need to consult your doctor for diagnosis and treatment.

ISBN 0-615-11444-X

Dedication

This book is dedicated to all those suffering people who've looked to me for help for their facial pain. I appreciate their trust and all the friendships I formed over the past two decades. My prayer is that more would have been helped. A day doesn't pass when I don't think of some . . .of several, who still suffer. I also dedicate this book to my staff, most of whom have been with me for more than 15 years. They are so kind and compassionate towards our patients. They truly minister to every one, each other, and to me. Most importantly, I dedicate this book to my Savior and Lord, Jesus Christ. He walks with me and talks with me. Every discovery I've made has been through the guidance of His Holy Spirit. God does all the healing . . . the doctor just sends the bill. *"Beloved, I pray that in all respects you may prosper and be in good health, just as your soul prospers."* 3 John 2

Foreword

Persons with facial pain face an array of diagnoses and treatments that are at times appropriate and at times inappropriate. This book educates the reader to the causes of facial pain and guides the reader through the usual treatments of facial pain with an uncanny ability to relate in everyday terminology.

Dr. Shankland is a leader in the world of diagnosis and treatment of facial pain. He has very few peers at his level of practice. This book is written out of his compassion for the patient in pain and more specifically chronic facial pain. Health care practitioners who treat chronic pain patients usually feel lead to do so by a higher power. This is more than evident with Dr. Shankland.

Most health care providers are well trained in acute pain treatment. The average health care provider does not feel comfortable seeing chronic pain patients. There is a void in the training of most health care professionals in the diagnosis and treatment of chronic pain, which is evidenced by the difficulty that the medical community has with treatment of this group of patients. The health care provider must spend countless hours of post-doctoral education to become competent in the diagnosis and treatment of the chronic pain patient. Dr. Shankland has traveled this road and has emerged as one of the premier practitioners treating facial pain today. This book will be known as "the book" to read for the person or family member of a person suffering with facial pain.

H. Clifton Simmons III, D.D.S.

Assistant Clinical Professor, Vanderbilt University College of Medicine, Department of Dentistry

President, American Academy of Craniofacial Pain, (2000 - 2002)

Diplomate, American Board of Craniofacial Pain

Diplomate, American Board of Orofacial Pain

Diplomate, American Academy of Pain Management

Acknowledgments

While a dental student at The Ohio State University, I studied under a very strict, yet understanding professor, Dr. Richard Huffman. He demanded the best from me at all times. I continued to study with him after graduation. He also became my good friend and humbled me when he once told a group of doctors, when asked about my philosophies on facial pain, said: "It's time for the professor to listen to his student." I'll never forget Dr. Huffman's influence on my life.

In 1982, I met Dr. Edwin Ernest of Montgomery, Alabama. Dr. Ernest has probably made more significant contributions to the area of orofacial pain than any other single person. He trained me, discipled me in orofacial pain and as a brother in Christ, and became one of my best friends. If I ever contribute anything to mankind concerning orofacial pain, it will be as a direct result of Dr. Ernest's influence upon my life.

I also wish to thank John Negulesco, Ph.D., for his encouragement and friendship. Dr. Negulesco was my advisor when I returned to graduate school. He took a chance accepting such an old student (I was 39). He cultivated my burning desire to explore the human body and was the one faculty member of the Department of Cell Biology, Neurobiology and Anatomy, The Ohio State University, who tolerated and supported my unusual hours and non-traditional approach to graduate school. John is also the finest educator and anatomist I've ever known.

I greatly appreciate Dr. Devin Starlanyl's chapter about Fibromyalgia. Dr. Starlanyl, a fibromyalgia sufferer herself, is probably the country's expert on this subject. Thank you, my dear friend, for your efforts.

Also, I'd like to thank my good friend Dr. James Boyd for his contribution to this book. Dr. Boyd is a dentist, an inventor, and a visionary. His device, the NTI, has changed the way we look at the cause and treatment of headache pain. Soon, the foundations of migraine treatment will also be shaken, because of his invention. Thanks, Jim.

As in my first book, I wish to thank my mother, Lorna Shankland. She always has been, and continues to be, my greatest cheerleader. Thanks, Mom.

I'm very appreciative of James Downard. As one of my patients, Jim has become my very best friend and my writing coach.

I also want to thank Doug Little, M. Div., Ph. D., and Lawrence Schlak, M. Div., Ph.D., for their wonderful advice concerning chapter two. Both of these men are former pastors; Dr. Little, a clinical psychologist, is a professor as Ashland Theological Seminary and Dr. Schlak, is a neuropsychologist for the State of Kentucky.

Thanks also go to my sister, Lisa, for her support and encouragement all these years. You know what I'm thinking!

I also wish to thank and praise my wonderful staff: Sherry, Jan, Kay, Karen, Melissa, Judy, Karan and Carrie. They are very patient with their eccentric boss.

I couldn't have complete this book without help from my editor, Terri Kelly.

My thoughts and efforts are directed to you, the reader. My prayer is that you'll learn something which may help relieve you or a loved one from the ravages of facial pain.

Table of Contents

Introduction

I wrote this book as a follow-up to *TMJ: Its Many Faces.* Even with the outstanding reception the first book received, I felt more information needed to be written for the general public. Billions of dollars are spent each year for health care, much for the diagnosis of pain. Pain sufferers will do and pay anything for some hope of relief. Unfortunately, insurance companies don't share such enthusiasm for pain relief. And it's going to get worse, at least in the United States. Because most doctors both don't understand nor pursue the numerous causes of pain, the medical profession won't demand reasonable payment from insurance companies for adequate pain treatment. It's funny to see how doctors and insurance executives alike change their attitudes when a loved one is in pain!

In 1983, I conducted a survey of 135 consecutive pain patients. We discovered that our office was the 6th, on average, to be consulted for orofacial pain problems. For one lady from Kentucky, I was her 31st doctor. Can you imagine that? I've also been the 29th doctor for one lady from Tennessee.

Two common denominators soon became apparent from that survey: The doctors apparently didn't listen about the patients' pain complaints; and, the doctors often didn't believe the patients' complaints. These commentaries on the medical and dental professions are sad. What's even worse is many doctors, regardless of degree, don't even believe in many pain syndromes. How can this be? Many doctors don't believe in pain disorders which weren't taught when they were in school and residency programs. That's awful arrogant because so much knowledge concerning pain has been discovered in recent years, many years after these so-called experts graduated.

I've been fortunate enough to be directly involved in the discovery and/or research of several pain disorders, none of which were known even as late as 1980. For a doctor to deny validity in a pain disorder not taught to him in school is like a pastor not believing in heaven or hell. It just doesn't make sense. It's intellectual suicide. I see suffering people every day. They're just like you and me, but unfortunately, for any number of reasons, they have an extra burden to carry: pain. Perhaps that's why I'm so cynical about my colleagues who refuse to believe these people are suffering.

Here's an example. This lady from California, sent this conversation with God just to demonstrate to me her extent of suffering:

> Oh Lord, Lord Jesus, why me? I have suffered long enough, yet I hold on hoping you will guide me to help. I have lost all my loved ones and stand alone with you by my side. Mom always told me to trust in the Lord, and take my troubles to you. I have those that love me and pray for me daily, but the pain is so horrible. It's so hard to keep believing that there will be a day when this horrible nerve will stop invading my mouth so that I can sing in church and pray with others out loud. It hurts so bad Lord. Please don't misunderstand my plea, as I know that so many are suffering with all kinds of pain. But Lord Jesus I know I could endure this so much easier and longer if it wasn't in my mouth. Forgive me for thinking bad thoughts, about not wanting to live, if I have to live with this every waking hour. So many times I think of just ending this pain, and joining you . . . I just keep on having faith that someone will believe me and help me through you. I ask your guidance and faith in the power of prayer. In Jesus' name . . . Amen
> Betty L (used with permission)

See why I felt this book was needed? Although severe, this dear lady isn't unusual. There are many people like this. Most doctors and insurance companies don't want to deal with them, so the suffering is magnified.

In this book, I've revisited the subjects of Pain and Neuralgia Inducing Cavitational Osteonecrosis (NICO). We've learned more about both these subjects since my first book was published. I included new and more in-depth material about pain, one subject that truly binds us all together. In addition, I've written the chapter on NICO both for the public and for health professionals. This horrible disorder of dead bone plagues so many, especially those with facial involvement. Subjects such as Odontalgia (tooth pain) and Burning Mouth Syndrome are presented, describing causes and successful forms of therapy. In addition, controversial, yet scientifically valid material is presented concerning the systemic effects of periodontal disease. Dr. James Boyd has presented some revolutionary information on bruxism and the treatment of this disorder. Lastly, I hope the tone of this book will be encouraging. Most pain conditions, if diagnosed correctly, can be helped. Without Divine intervention, many pain syndromes can't be cured, but most can be significantly improved.

CHAPTER One

Face The Pain

Consider the human face. In a sense, its musculature contorts whenever we eat, drink, speak, smile, yawn, laugh and if fortunate, enjoy a kiss. These distortions are normal for us as we proceed through our daily activities. In fact, we consider such facial alterations as normal and rarely do these changes in one's facial expressions catch our attention. Only extremes of joy, anger, excitement and grief proclaim themselves in what we'd consider as distortions of human the face.

The face is the organ of emotion. We constantly read facial expressions to understand what others are feeling. Our faces contain and convey powerful clues, almost like a dynamic canvas, one in which emotions are drawn vividly, then suddenly erased, only to be redrawn in a new expression an instant later. Our identity is captured in our facial features, and our eyes reveal important truths about us, even those we would prefer to conceal.

> *Our identity is captured in our facial features, and our eyes reveal important truths about us, even those we would prefer to conceal.*

While the face is the organ of emotion, it's also much more. The face is an important channel of identity. Friends and acquaintances can recognize us before a word is spoken. Our face develops as we do, from infancy, into adulthood, crossing into middle age, and finally into the senior years--always retaining features prominent in childhood.

The face is also our most powerful channel of nonverbal communication. We encode messages in our own facial expressions, and we simultaneously decode the faces of the people around us as quickly as 165 thousandths of a second! In even the most simple interaction, our attention naturally gravitates to the face, seeking to read some of the vital information we know is written there.

We constantly monitor the face because it provides vital clues to an impressive variety of possibilities: attraction; whether a person likes or dislikes us; the complexity of emotions; identity; age; humor; and a person's regional and even national background.

Physically, our face is the most important human art object. Cosmetics, coloration, hair length and style, and other qualities all figure in perceptions of physical attractiveness. People can even decide to permanently modify this most personal art object by piercing facial structures or through plastic surgery. The normal human face is possibly the most beautifully perfect structure in all of creation.

At Face Value

Acute or immediate pain and chronic pain are vastly different (see Chapter 2). Most of us, whether in the health sciences or not, can recognize the facial characteristics of someone in acute pain:

- Pressing the lips together, especially at the corners
- Parting the lips
- Turning the head
- Lowering the brow
- Perspiration
- Paleness
- Raising the upper lip/nose wrinkling
- Jaw drooping
- Eyes closing or frequently blinking

If you've been with someone recently injured, you know these are universal characteristics of acute pain. Current research supports the idea that these acute pain characteristics occur in both infants and adults, at least in Western cultures. **But what about the facial appearance of one suffering with chronic pain?**

Chronic pain sufferers' facial expressions are different from those of acute pain sufferers. Emotional expressions of acute pain are virtually absent in those with chronic pain. If you saw these people in a department store, they'd look perfectly normal, and that's one of the problems of chronic pain: the sufferers don't look like they're in pain. However, if you spend any time talking with chronic pain sufferers, their facial expressions rarely change, almost frozen no matter what the situation or topic under discussion. These are the people I see every day in my office. On average, I'm the sixth doctor they've consulted for their complaints of pain, so they're hardly excited to see me. They often come into the office with a spouse or parent, emotionless and quiet. The lack of facial expressions betrays them.

> *Rarely changing facial expressions, chronic pain sufferers look sober, stern or serious all the time. And those with orofacial pain are even worse.*

We're told the eyes are the windows to the soul. Believe me, you can see deep into the soul of one with chronic, orofacial pain. They may say everything's alright when asked, but their eyes betray them. An observant doctor watches his patient's eyes for many clues, especially for clues about pain and emotional suffering.

Rarely changing facial expressions, chronic pain sufferers look sober, stern or serious all the time. And those with orofacial pain are even worse. Even the slightest smile often triggers their pain symptoms. They don't go outside except when they absolutely have to because wind, rain, and even the heat of the sun may stimulate their pain.

Because of the anatomical complexity and due to our deeply seated emotional relationships to our face, pain in this area of the body is often perceived as being worse than if the same type and intensity of pain affected another location. Just looking at these patients, their facial countenance says, "I'm frustrated." "I'm depressed." "I'm ready to give up."

Facial pain frequently radiates into the head, thus producing headache pain as well. If the headache pain is severe enough to drive the patient to any type of doctor, he may be misdiagnosed as having migraine headaches, and the initial source of pain in the face may be totally over-looked.

There are numerous causes of facial pain, many of which we'll explore in this book. Probably the most encouraging words you can read are: There is hope for your pain! In most cases, there is an answer, just don't give up.

References

1. **Halgren E, Raij T, Marinkovic K, Jousmaki V, Hari R**: *Cognitive Response Profile of the Human Fusiform Face Area as Determined by MEG.* Cereb Cortex 2000 Jan;10(1):69-81.

2. **Raij T**: *Patterns of brain activity during visual imagery of letters.* J Cogn Neurosci 1999; 11:282-99.

3. **Craig KD, Patrick CJ**: *Facial expression during induced pain.* J Pers Soc Psychol 1985;48:1080-1091.

4. **Prkachin PM**: *The consistency of facial expressions of pain: a comparison across modalities.* Pain 1992;51:297-306.

5. **LeResche L, Dworkin SF**: *Facial expression accompanying pain.* Soc Sci Med 1984;19:1325-1330.

6. **Malatesta CZ, Jonas R, Izard CE**: *The relation between low facial expressivity during emotional arousal and somatic symptoms.* Br J Med Psychol 1987;60:169-180.

CHAPTER Two

Concept of Pain

"Physical pain is not a simple affair of an impulse, traveling at a fixed rate along a nerve. It is the result of a conflict between a stimulus and the whole individual."   Rene Leriche

The concept of pain has captivated mankind since the beginning of recorded history. Pain commands human beings to behave in ways otherwise avoided. Pain may even be an ally of the sufferer, an excuse to avoid unpleasant tasks or situations when convenient. Realize, too, that pain is a private experience. We can only measure the behavior or expression of those in pain, not the pain itself.

Like pain, suffering is also a private experience. Both human beings and animals have the ability to perceive pain. Animals scream, howl, or run away from a painful stimulus. In human beings, however, pain is far more complex. Often, we can't scream or even run from the source of pain. Further, each person reacts differently to the same stimulus of pain. But why?

Private experience. We can only measure the behavior of those in pain, not the pain itself.

The real question is: What is pain? Each has his description of this nebulous term. Say "pain" and we imagine hitting our fingers with a hammer or slamming our hand in a car door. Some of us think of the pain of defeat or the pain after the break-up of a relationship. Obviously, pain can have many meanings, but which one, if any, is correct?

Although our English language may be the most flexible, changeable language today, it fails sometimes by not being sufficiently specific. For example, consider the word *love*. Which of the following is correct?

- I love my family
- I love my friends
- I love NASCAR racing
- I love my dogs (all 9 of them!)

They're all correct! Pain is an excellent example of how English employs one word a variety of ways and for doctors and patients alike, this simple word causes much confusion.

Latin and Greek have several words for pain. Unlike English, these ancient languages have specific words for specific types of pain (for example, physical pain, the pain of hunger, mental anguish, sickness, and suffering).

By contrast, English uses just one word, *pain*, to mean physical pain, suffering, anguish, sickness, etc. This apparent communication problem concerning the meaning of pain is now a worldwide phenomena because English is the recognized language of science.

A definition of the word pain might clarify this issue. But that's not as easy as we might think. Do we mean pain or suffering? Are they the same?

Pain: An unpleasant experience, which we associate with tissue damage or perceived tissue damage.

Researchers have attempted to define pain for thousands of years. A simple definition of pain is: "An unpleasant experience associated with tissue damage." But tissue damage doesn't always have to occur for one to experience pain. An example: phantom limb pain or pain perceived in an arm or leg that was amputated years earlier. Also, we've been created with a great capacity to experience and convey emotions. So, a major difficulty in defining pain has been the confusion of physical complaints with emotional disturbances, both of which English speakers call pain. So, we're back where we started, attempting to define the word pain more precisely.

Combining the ideas of physical pain and emotional suffering, we might define pain as: "An unpleasant experience, which we associate with tissue damage or perceived tissue damage." We'll use this definition of pain throughout this book.

Types of Pain

Basically, there are two general categories of pain: acute and chronic. Acute pain is limited to the first few hours, days, or at most and depending upon classic definitions, up to six months. However, current research shows us that any painful condition, persisting longer that two weeks, will develop the characteristics of chronic pain.

Acute Pain

Acute pain is a time-limited experience. It's caused by tissue damage. This immediate type of pain (for example, a fractured bone, a laceration, or a broken tooth) causes fear and anxiety in the injured person. Usually, the greater the anxiety, the greater the reaction to the painful stimulus and therefore, the more display of pain behavior (see below).

When we are injured, our nervous system informs us of the exact location of the damaged tissue. Our body reacts by performing a series of physiological processes in an attempt to avoid any further injury and to survive. The physiological series of events following an injury are actually defense mechanisms.

Ever twisted or sprained your ankle? You probably noticed an immediate severe, sharp, bright pain informing you of the exact location of the injury. Your heart rate and blood pressure increased, and you may have even become nauseated. If the injury was severe enough, you also became faint. You had to sit down. You had no choice.

A few minutes after the injury, you noticed a dull, throbbing, deep and aching pain replacing the sharp pain. Swelling most likely began quickly, and standing on the painful ankle reproduced your sharp pain.

Anxiety and possibly fear developed as you realized that you were injured. Your face showed the classic signs of acute pain: a furrowed brow, eyes squeezed shut, your teeth clenched, and the telltale facial grimace. Every human being, no matter what his or her ethnic, racial, or religious background, exhibits these classic reactions to acute injury. However, past the initial reaction to injury, people exhibit wide variations in how they manage both acute and chronic pain, should the later develop.(see below).

Chronic Pain

Persisting long after the apparent healing of injured tissues, chronic pain is both frustrating and can be quite costly. Like acute pain, chronic pain has emotional characteristics. The longer the pain persists, the greater the probability that a depressed mood and fear will arise. The injured person becomes irritable and often irrational in his or her search for pain relief. If the pain continues, the sufferer may develop specific pain behaviors and coping mechanisms (see below). While the classic facial grimace of acute pain is absent, chronic pain patients exhibit a depressed, melancholy appearance, both with their facial expressions and with their body posture.

> *While the classic facial grimace of acute pain is absent, chronic pain patients exhibit a depressed, melancholy appearance, both with their facial expressions and with their body posture.*

Chronic pain has a language all its own, often described as stabbing like a knife or an ice pick. There may be intense pressure along with the pain. Unlike acute pain, the exact source of chronic pain is often difficult to locate.

It's interesting to watch a patient describe his or her pain. The acute pain patient is often excited, animated, and able to locate the exact source of the pain, but chronic pain patients often describe their pain symptoms in a subdued, relaxed, almost distracted manner. Unlike the acute pain patient, chronic pain sufferers often change the subject or are easily distracted when reporting their present pain history.

For example, if you're stung by a wasp, your behavior (both voluntary and involuntary) is predictable, whether you're a college football player, a member of English nobility, or a tribesman in South America. Your behavior won't matter much because you know both the sting and pain will last only briefly, and you'll recover soon. But if you're diagnosed with trigeminal neuralgia (Chapter 3), and the doctor says you may suffer with pain the rest of your life, the situation is far more serious and you'll develop behavior patterns to prevent the severe facial pain from totally dominating your life. If you successfully alter your behavior, you'll raise your level of pain tolerance.

Further, depression is quite common with the chronic pain patient possibly due to the persistence of pain, causing the fear of loss of control. Many prescription pain medications can produce or enhance depression. Obsessed with a pursuit of recovery and preoccupation with pain symptoms, these people develop worse or pathological behaviors.

A final comment about chronic pain: The sufferers are often treated in such a fashion, which, according to Dr. Norman Marcus in his book, *Freedom from Chronic Pain*, creates a series of factors that he calls the *Seven Ds*. Dr. Marcus writes about chronic pain in general, but these seven principles certainly apply, with a few modifications, to orofacial pain:

• **Doctor shopping.** Patients travel from doctor to doctor, office to office, and clinic to clinic in search of help for their chronic pain. In a study conducted in 1983, I was the 6th physician, on average, consulted for the relief of chronic pain. For one lady, I was her 31st doctor; another, her 19th. Such doctor shopping is understandable, but unfortunately, costly and frequently dangerous, as these patients are desperate and will do anything for even partial relief of their pain. I've noticed in my practice that the Internet has helped to reduce the numbers of doctors and clinics in one's wake as they wander, looking for answers for their pain.

• **Dollars.** In addition to feeling terrible, chronic pain sufferers spend tremendous amounts of money and generally, they receive very little help (and compassion) from insurance companies. Not only do these patients spend thousands of dollars, but emotionally there's also a cost. My problem is trying to convince a patient, who has spent count-less dollars and has been disappointed so many times, that I might be able to help. Without knowing me, I'm just one more in a long line of doctors. I certainly understand the reluctance to try once more with me.

• **Drugs.** Virtually every chronic pain patient I see has collected more drugs than most drug stores. This may be an exaggeration, but chronic pain patients do accumulate many different medications because they've seen so many different doctors, all of whom have their own preferred medicines. Also, if you suffer with chronic pain, you're forced to consume more and more of the same medication because your tolerance builds up over time. You may become dependent due to no fault of your own. I term this *supervised neglect* and like so many doctors, I too, am guilty of this with some of my pa-tients. Unless you're plagued with chronic pain, you can't understand what I'm saying.

• **Doubt.** A common and frustrating problem which al-most all chronic pain patients experience is doubt. Doctors, unable to find the cause of pain, cast doubt and influence the patient's family members. Soon, the patient himself doubts if he has real pain or not. If you're in this situation, realize that doctors have an ego problem if they can't find the cause of your pain. We're taught to be methodical, observe every detail, and if we can't discover the source of pain, then maybe it's in the patient's head. Some of my colleagues, who would never consider treating chronic pain patients, often ask if most of my patients are crazy. I usually reply: "They are now after going through the medical red tape time and time again!"

• **Disuse.** We all want to avoid pain, so when we hurt, we avoid activities which might reproduce or intensify our pain complaints. Unfortunately, disuse produces atrophy (wasting-away) of muscles, bones and strength. Weakness occurs. Once this happens, we can experience a secondary type of pain and aching when engaging in any physical activities. It's unfortunate, but doctors usually recommend chronic pain patients rest, stay in bed, and refrain from physical activities, ultimately making the pain condition worse.

• **Depression.** Chronic pain in general, but disuse specifically, produce depression. You feel as if you're not human, no longer valuable to your family, or life may no longer be worth living. If you feel like this, realize you're mistaken. Scientific breakthroughs in the management of chronic pain are coming faster than ever before. I'm very encouraged by what's happened in the last few years in the field of chronic pain, and you, too need to be encouraged. Hang onto hope!

• **Disability.** Chronic pain suffering often leads to disability. But even disabled people can lead happy, productive lives. Often, just changing your job or lifestyle can decrease the effects of your condition. Far too often, doctors and family members alike develop a prejudicial attitude against disabled pain patients, often thinking of these people as lazy and trying to milk the system just to obtain disability payments.

All of us need to work hard to dispel the terrible attitudes about and against sufferers of chronic pain. In over 23 years of practice, I've met at most, two or three patients who wanted to be labeled as pain patients. Those miserable people had a psychological disorder termed Munchausen's syndrome, a disorder termed a *factitious disorder*. These patients deliberately mislead others into thinking they (or their children - Munchausen by proxy) have serious medical or psychological problems, often resulting in extraordinary numbers of medication trials, diagnostic tests, hospitalizations, and even surgery that they know aren't really needed. In short, factitious disorders involve disease forgery. Why someone would engage in such behavior is difficult to understand, but I've seen this a couple of times, especially when marital conflict is great. Munchausen patients often:

• Feign (fake) illnesses

• Falsify lab results
  (e.g., by adding blood or protein to a urine specimen)

• Aggravate existing medical problems
  (e.g., by manipulating a wound so it doesn't heal)

• Cause an actual illness
  (e.g., by injecting themselves or their child
  with bacteria to cause a raging infection)

Doctors must be aware of this type of patient, but usually, we aren't. All the medicine, physical therapy or surgery will not help these people until they receive psychological counseling first.

Pain Behavior

How can we know the extent to which one is experiencing pain? We've all heard of the soldier who, after being seriously wounded, still managed to perform an act of remarkable bravery without any concern for pain until the danger passed. What about the person who appears to experience severe pain sitting in the dental chair even though the doctor has just touched a tooth and nothing more?

In contrast, there are dental patients who allow any number of procedures to be performed without any use of local anesthetic and never flinch or blink an eye.

A personal note. There's one old gentleman I'll never forget. In the first couple of years I was in private practice, I made house calls for Hospice, a caring and invaluable program—actually a ministry of sorts—caring for the terminally ill in their homes in the company of their family members. Called to this elderly gentleman's home because he had an abscessed tooth needing immediate treatment, I examined him and recommended extraction of the tooth. He agreed with one stipulation: that I use no local anesthetic! Most people get sick when they need a tooth removed even when numbed with more than adequate anesthesia. Imagine how I felt, a young dentist, making one of my first house calls, and challenged to perform a surgical procedure without giving the patient an anesthetic? Guess who was shaking and perspiring through the entire procedure? The old man just laughed and never flinched as I surgically removed his abscessed tooth.

Obviously, there was actual, not perceived, tissue damage when I removed the old guy's tooth; but one would never have known it–and he certainly wasn't going to admit feeling any pain whatsoever.

And then there's the huge professional football player who breaks into a cold sweat just shaking the dentist's hand. This is the guy who requires a tremendous amount of anesthetic and then, often faints during a routine dental procedure.

What's the difference between these people? As human beings, we all have the same types of nerve receptors, which are capable of being stimulated. But why the wide range of diversity between the perception of pain among people? Keep in mind that pain is a private experience. We can only measure the behavior of those in pain and not the pain itself.

Definition of Pain Behavior

Probably the best definition for pain behavior is: "Anything a person says or does to reflect the presence of tissue damage."

No matter what the pain syndrome may be, pain behavior has the following characteristics:

Pain behavior is anything a person says or does to reflect the presence of tissue damage.

• **It's real.** Being a private experience, we can never know what a pain sufferer is actually feeling or sensing. We can only observe one's behavior to pain.

• **Pain behavior is measured subjectively.** We can measure one's pain: By the amount of medication he or she consumes; by reviewing responses in a pain diary, or by observing such activities as guarded movements, grimacing, rubbing painful areas, avoiding social and physical activities, moaning, avoiding sex, avoiding work, and sighing.

• **Pain behavior is influenced by immediate and anticipated consequences of that behavior.** An old Chinese proverb often applies: "Pain is not good without an audience." Many people who suffer with chronic pain syndromes develop behaviors, which at times, are used for the sufferer's advantage, and often in the presence of other people.

Pain behavior frequently leads to secondary gain such as:

- Sympathy

- Affection

- Attention from others

- Relief of responsibilities

- Power

- Control

Pain behaviors fall into two categories: (1) innate (or, reflexive) and (2) learned. Withdrawal, moaning, rubbing, and certain facial expressions are probably genetically determined reflexes initiated by tissue damage. Other reactions to pain are most likely learned, partly by children mimicking adults and partially by being rewarded for behavior deemed appropriate (being cuddled, receiving attention, not having to perform certain physical activities, or even receiving gifts from parents or grandparents).

An Example of Pain Behavior

Observing pain behaviors in my office is quite interesting. I may see 35 or 40 patients a day, most of whom are in pain or have recently experienced pain. I recall a recent episode in which, with a reception room and office full of patients, a woman in her late 30s, with no appointment, came bursting into the office, moaning and crying uncontrollably. She was accompanied by her husband and her 18-month-old daughter. Obviously, this disrupted the office and caused a great deal of stress among the office staff, not to mention concern among those in the reception room waiting to see me–some for the first time. She was wailing, the baby was crying, and her husband was not the least bit happy.

My receptionist immediately ushered her into an examining room, ahead of others who had appointments (rewarding her loud and disruptive behavior). I was very busy, performing an intricate surgical procedure for an out-of-state patient. I could hear her noises—Lord, who couldn't! After carefully placing the last suture, I hurried down the hall to attend to her, as her noises had escalated absurdly. When I walked into the room, upon seeing me, she ceased all moaning and crying, almost on cue. My assistant was amazed. I wasn't.

My assistant had unwittingly validated the woman's behavior by dropping everything she was doing to attend to this lady (further rewarding her behavior) in front of the husband (more reward and validation of her pain for her benefit, almost proving to her husband that she really had a painful disorder and he should be ashamed for being upset with her). There really was tissue damage, but, by exhibiting such behavior, she was able to magnify and use her pain syndrome for her benefits . . . whatever they may have been.

You're probably thinking that I'm cruel and uncaring, and just the type of doctor you'd love to see. Well, I do care, but I don't appreciate manipulation, especially when others in pain were patiently and quietly waiting to be seen.

What did I do? After I spoke quietly to her about her inappropriate display of pain, she remained quiet and surprisingly composed. She still complained of severe, uncontrollable pain. I quickly injected the painful site with saline solution and not local anesthetic! Guess what happened? Within seconds, all pain ceased and her behavior became perfectly normal and socially acceptable. Had I used a local anesthetic to numb the painful area, the effects of the anesthetic would have taken several minutes, not seconds, to take effect.

See what I'm trying to say about pain behavior? This lady's pain worked well for her in the presence of her audience. For her, "Pain *was* good with an audience."

Factors Which Effect Pain Behavior

Cellular membranes are so intricate in their anatomy and functions that our most advanced computers couldn't begin to design such structures. And nerve cells (neurons) have additional complexity. Even though each of us is equipped with the same types of nerve cells, many other factors influence our perception of pain. Anatomically, we're all the same, but psychologically, we're vastly different.

With all of us having common anatomical structures, numerous factors influence our reactions to pain, many of which are listed below. Remember, pain is a private experience, but pain behavior is greatly determined by our cultural and social backgrounds.

Relationship to Therapist

Psychological factors influence the way we handle a potentially painful experience. A relationship with the therapist is one. If you know and trust the doctor, nurse, or therapist, then chances are your reactions to a painful experience will be quite different than if you had no relationship with a new dentist or an emergency room physician. A relationship with the doctor gives one a sense of comfort and assurance, even in the most stressful situations. If you don't believe this, just ask any woman who's given birth if she'd like a strange doctor to deliver her baby.

Family Influences

Perhaps in your family, pain was ridiculed. Pain was "All in your head." Maybe your parents (because of their parents and other influences) taught you that to show pain demonstrated weakness, especially in public. In fact, our society rather admires this stoic attitude. Think of action movies. The hero is often seriously injured and yet, rarely exhibits any reaction to pain and continues to function in an almost "super-human" form. This myth and some parental attitudes can produce severe guilt in a person who genuinely has been injured. We're told such lies as, "It can't hurt," or "Real men don't cry." As I grow older I'm learning that real men do cry.

Ethnic or Cultural Influences

Have you even attended an Italian wedding? What a celebration and display of happiness and anticipation for the couple being married. The food, the drink, the dancing! Better not plan on leaving early. The party will probably last for hours.

By contrast, being of European, Protestant decent, my wedding was short and sweet–the way I like it. We had a small reception, with no dancing or music, just food and talk with the guests. The wedding and reception lasted only two and-a-half hours, about two hours too long for me!

Just as ethnic differences can affect weddings, they can affect reaction to pain. Those raised in large, extended families generally exhibit an exaggerated response to pain.

One researcher published in the *Journal of Social Issues* a report about specific examples of cultural differences. He discovered that Old Americans (those Americans who families have lived in North America for many generations) have an accepting, matter-of-fact attitude towards pain and their expression of pain. On the other hand, individuals of Jewish and Italian descent tend to be quite vocal in their complaints about pain and openly seek support and sympathy. The underlying attitudes of these latter two groups appear to be different. Jewish individuals tend to be concerned with the meaning and ramifications of their pain, whereas the Italians usually express a desire for immediate relief of pain.

I'm not implying that such behavioral display is wrong or even inappropriate. Who am I to pronounce what's socially acceptable? In fact, psychosocially, such behavior is important within individual communities. In some cultures, exaggerated pain behavior is normal and expected. But we also have to realize that such ethnic factors greatly influence pain-driven behavior.

Consider those staunch, Calvinistic Lutheran or Presbyterian families, demanding strong determination and non-emotional public displays of behavior. Religious influences aside, these folks generally exhibit little emotion, whether as reaction to pain or celebrations, such as weddings or funerals. Does this behavior imply that these people are less joyous or experience less sorrow because they don't publicly exhibit such emotions. Not at all!

By the way, the disruptive lady whom I described above, was a member of an ethnic group known for wild and noisy public displays of emotions. In that context, her behavior was not that unusual. As the doctor charged with determining a proper diagnosis and subsequent treatment, I was seriously challenged. I needed to attempt to ignore much of her behavior and focus on discovering the actual source of her pain.

Past Experiences

"The bigger they are, the harder they fall." Those of us in pain management find it comical that huge, well-conditioned football players, who engage in violent physical contacts in a game, are often terrified when they visit the dentist. In contrast, small, frail women give birth without any anesthetic or sedative. What's the difference?

In the light of past experiences, anticipation of pain causes great apprehension. The huge football player, visiting the dentist, knows that the doctor wants only to help. We sadly realize, at times, elimination of a pathological problem requires the infliction of some pain. If one has been hurt in the past while undergoing dental care, a great chance exists that past experiences will influence one's reaction to health care.

Age of Patient

Studies with bone cancer and juvenile arthritis suggest that people experience greater pain with increasing age, especially as one approaches adulthood. Some anatomists have observed that children seem to exhibit a lesser display of pain, perhaps, because of yet undeveloped somatosensory pathways (sensory pathways to the brain). Some psychologists believe children's pain perception may be manipulated more easily than in older children or adults. Both views may contain a bit of truth.

Also, children seem to express less pain behavior possibly because they've not yet learned acceptable social responses to painful conditions. They're troubled by visible injuries such as a cut finger or the sight of blood.

Unfortunately, this apparent lesser display of pain behavior in children permits adults to dismiss or ignore pain complaints of children. A classic case is headache pain. How often have you seen a television advertisement for headache medication in which a child was featured as the headache sufferer? Further, when was the last time you even heard of a child suffering with a headache?

Convincing parents and doctors alike that children are no different than adults, that they develop painful conditions, has increased the number of children I see in my office. These kids are really great, and they usually heal much faster than older folks, say, a 25 or 30 year old!

Take children seriously when they complain of pain. As with most embarrassing situations, children are generally brutally honest, even concerning pain.

Religious Beliefs

Religious beliefs may greatly influence one's reaction to pain. Scientific studies show religious patients report significantly lower levels of pain, but are no less likely to report pain. Psychologically, some doctors dismiss this negative correlation as denial or unrealistic stoicism. If this denial lessens perceived pain, then this type of denial must be a desirable goal.

Maybe the scientists should realize that prayer does change things!

Maybe the scientists should realize that prayer does change things!

On the other hand, what if prayer about a specific pain problem doesn't change things? What if the gnawing pain is more recognizable than the calm of God?

Many of my patients are committed Christians. As a fellow Believer, I'm saddened by some of the brethrens' unrealistic attitudes towards disease and pain. Self-imposed guilt (see next section) and feeling unworthy of healing are common, but the ones who dismay me most are the religious who refuse to accept painful conditions as a consequence of life. They quote all the favorite scriptures and proclaim they aren't going to receive their condition in spite of the objective findings and their subjective complaints. "Doctor, pray for me. I know God will heal me. I don't need medicine, 'cause God's healing me. I refuse to accept this disease."

I pray and believe, but I also know God heals through men and women, medicine and surgery. I've seen dramatic demonstrations of divine healing through, and in spite of, doctors, but I've also seen those not healed, for whatever the reason. Jesus never condemned doctors. Luke was a physician and Jesus Himself said, "It is not those who are healthy who need a physician but those who are sick." (Mat 9:12)

I've heard my favorite Bible teacher, Dr. Charles Stanley, say many times, "When you're in the midst of pain, ask God what He's teaching you through that experience." I agree and try to encourage my patients to both pray and believe God will heal, but also, try to learn what they might in the midst of the pain.

Guilt

Some pain sufferers view pain as punishment and develop feelings of guilt, or, as Wall and Jones report in their book, *Defeating Pain*, intensify guilt feelings if they already exist. In some cases, there are objective reasons for a consciousness of guilt. One may have caused a motor vehicle accident by careless driving. Or, a child might be injured because the supposed attentive father was preoccupied with a sporting event on television. Another may blame his cancer or coronary heart disease on years of heavy smoking or unwise eating. In most cases, however, guilt is imaginary. Unfortunately, people develop cancer or have heart problems regardless of habits.

Guilt is a useless reaction to pain because such self-imposed feelings fail to remove the pain. Worse than useless, guilt may be harmful. The sufferer dwells on guilt, punishing himself, which serves only to cause more sensations of pain, reducing the level of pain tolerance.

If admitting guilt and saying, "I'm sorry" does no good, or if forgiveness of oneself and by others isn't ensuing, then guilt is very influential. A vicious cycle develops: Profession of guilt leads to obsessive contemplation about the guilt, leading to anxiety which, in turn, produces more guilt and heightens anxiety. These patients have little chance of learning to live with their pain.

Anxiety

Anxious patients generally display exaggerated pain behavior. Fear of anticipated pain, progression of a disease (whether actual or imagined), deformity, disappointing family members, or even the imagined fear of death greatly aggravate pain behavior.

The fear of loss of control of one's life affects pain behavior. This is especially true if one fears losing a job, workers' compensation benefits, or being denied treatment by an insurance company. They become desperate, panicky, and oftentimes, irrational.

Anxiety heightens arousal to environmental clues, causing patients to misinterpret any unusual sensation or feeling as a worsening of their condition. If a patient focuses on a potentially painful experience, he or she will tend to perceive pain more intensely than normal due to anxiety. In a clinical setting, we avoid the use of the word *pain* as much as possible. If a patient hears that magic word, his or her level of anxiety is heightened.

Anxiety heightens arousal to environmental clues, causing patients to misinterpret any unusual sensation or feeling as a worsening of their condition.

By contrast, we also know that distraction from pain reduces a patient's anxiety and thus, reduces his or hers reaction to pain. This is especially true if the pain is constant or rises slowly in intensity.

Anxious patients often exhibit the behavior of over-whelming pain, and when anxiety is severe and unrelieved, depression develops. The underlying causes of anxiety must to be addressed to have a chance for successful treatment of the physical pain. I often refer such patients to clinical psychologists, social workers, or trained counselors and pastors.

Self-Pity

The most common pattern of pain behavior is self-pity. These people tell everyone and give elaborate descriptions of their pain, providing running commentaries, often punctuated by crying, groaning and moaning. Family members mistake self-pity for depression, but unlike the former, depression sufferers tend to remain silent.

In western society, we regard self-pity as irritating and it angers us. However, this disapproval is resented by the self-pitier. To him, his pain is real and he feels a right to feel sorry for himself. He may develop a continual concentration on his pain problems, which only serves to reinforce the self-pity. In a sick, mentally distorted manner, self-pity becomes pleasure and like most of life's pleasures, it may be further cultivated and become a way of life.

Wall and Jones write, "As the word implies, self-pity is an essentially selfish stance." The sufferer feels free – justified – to complain and demand that the world revolve around him. He can't be left alone. Someone always has to be with him, be within calling distance, and prepared to drop all activities to attend to the self-pitier. In a distorted manner, he enjoys being in control and the privilege of being short-tempered.

This person is a manipulator. He acts powerless, but with such behavior, he becomes the most powerful person in the family or organization. Take his pain away, he's power-less. Therefore, if proper treatment relieves his pain, he accepts his improved physical condition grudgingly, not gratefully like others.

Self-pity's caustic effects take their toll. Family members and associates, as well as the sufferer himself, are affected. Others feel sacrificed to the sufferer's demands, but he alienates himself from the affection and sympathy he seeks. He cries, "You don't love me" or "You hope I die." The targeted person of these proclamations denies them, but secretly feels some truth in them. Ultimately, relationships may end, further justifying, in the self-pitier's mind, his behavior.

A personal note. My first memorable encounter with a patient crippled with self-pity occurred several years ago. A patient was in the hospital at Ohio State. I was called to consult with the Department of Physical Medicine, and so, I examined this mid-aged lady and began treatment. Although she responded nicely, her attitude remained miserable. She complained and cried. She'd driven her family away and being in the hospital probably gave family members an emotional rest.

The day finally came when I discharged her from the hospital. Coincidentally, her husband selected the same day to serve her with divorce papers. Immediately, she cried and moaned and refused to leave the hospital, all the while, screaming at the nursing staff and me. Moments earlier, she was fine, but after the papers, too ill to leave. Her family couldn't leave the room or else she'd scream and moan even more.

She finally left the hospital pronounced well by me, but to her, still very ill. Her manipulation was rewarded with a withdrawal of the divorce papers. After all, in our society, we don't kick a dog when he's down, do we?

That's not the end of the story. A few weeks later, I, too received some papers. This lady, who objectively was improving until her husband attempted to challenge her command of the family, was now suddenly ill again. My reward? She sued me for negligence and malpractice. After all, according to her, had I been competent, she would have gotten better, been able to return home, and her husband and family would have placed her back in her position of authority, fueled by self-pity.

Fortunately the law suit was dropped when others quickly offered their stories to the lady's attorney concerning her selfish, bizarre control over everyone in her sphere of influence.

Placebo Effect

Never underestimate the effectiveness of placebos. In drug studies, subjects taking placebos (usually sugar or salt) report about a 35% to a 50% marked reduction of pain! Even more incredible: The more severe the pain, the more effective are placebos.

In addition, two placebo capsules are more effective than one. Large placebo capsules are better than smaller ones. Also, injected placebos are more effective than those swallowed.

Psychologically, much of the placebo effect arises from the therapist's enthusiasm and the patient's confidence in the therapist. Anatomically, many descending pathways travel from the brain, mostly unconscious, which greatly influence the ascending pathways which carry pain sensations from injured areas in the body to the brain.

Brain Filtering

In addition to these psychological and social factors, we also have a very important sensory suppression system: descending pathways from the brain to filter-out unnecessary stimuli.

To prove how influential descending control of the brain is, try this experiment: Try not to feel the chair you're sitting in. Don't feel your watchband, or the waistband of your underwear. Silly? Maybe, but see how our brains filter-out non-essential stimuli? To be honest, this filtering occurs in our spinal cord *and* by descending brain pathways. Now, our challenge is to "filter-out" pain like we filter out the feeling of our underwear!

A personal note. A former patient comes to mind. Years ago, I treated an elderly lady for a painful condition in her face. The family and I thought she exaggerated her pain behavior. I couldn't find any pathological cause or explanation for her symptoms. With her children's permission, I obtained some chocolate coated candies from a local discount store which looked like red, round pills but had no writing on the outside. I placed several of them in a pill envelope and instructed the lady to take one every six hours for the next 10 days. I told her that I was sure that they would relieve her pain. I cautioned her not to ever bite but always swallow each "pill." She did as I instructed and within a few days, her pain was totally gone, much to the relief of her children and me, the placebo doc.

Coping With Chronic Pain

As if the above factors didn't make pain behavior and pain management difficult enough, we human beings operate within the context of several different types of coping strategies. Some of the more common coping strategies are:

• **Seeking more information.** The rational or intellectual approach to handling pain is to learn as much as you can about your problem. Today, with the incredible Internet, patients frequently learn almost as much as the doctor. Armed with such knowledge, they often intimidate or even anger some doctors. I enjoy examining a patient who has taking time to investigate his or her possible problem.

• **Talking with others.** Psychologists call this shared concern. I sometimes call it, a sister's advice. There's nothing wrong with talking to others about your pain problems, but realize that even a trained person can't give accurate advice unless he or she has performed a thorough physical exam.

• **Laughing at the problem.** Many cope with painful conditions by making fun of the situation, almost denying any thought of the possible consequences. We sarcastic people rely on coping strategy . . . just ask my wife.

• **Forgetting,** putting the painful condition out of mind, or suppressing any thoughts about the current pain problem. At times, this may be denying that the problem exists, especially a terminal problem. At other times, stoics tend to "get on with life" and live with their pain.

- **Distracting themselves** by doing other things or involving themselves in outside activities. I often recommend this type of activity for those with pain. As you give to others, you tend to forget about your problems and oftentimes, life's problems are put into a truer perspective when you focus on others.

- **Confronting the pain problem,** actually taking firm or positive action based upon one's understanding of the condition. Taking responsibility is a healthy response to a painful problem. Unfortunately, confronting a painful condition sometimes leads to aggressive, unnecessary and irreversible medical procedures.

- **Accepting the painful condition.** Sometimes the sufferer attempts to find something advantageous about the painful hand life has dealt him or her.

- **Submitting to and accepting the inevitable,** whatever it may be. This fatalistic attitude often hinders treatment because the patient has resolved in his or her mind that, "What will be, will be."

- **Selecting alternative activities,** no matter how reckless or impractical, to divert attention away from the painful condition. This coping mechanism also often leads to irreparable and disfiguring surgical procedures which only serve to make the patient's pain worse. This attitude not only hinders treatment, but it's also responsible for diseases and injuries to progress.

- **Negotiating reasonable alternatives.** At times, negotiators manipulate others or family members to permit normally unacceptable behaviors to ease the painful condition.

- Reducing the stress of a pain disorder by **drinking, overeating,** or taking inappropriate quantities of pain medications. This is the hardest coping mechanism a doctor must face. Not only does the patient tend to lose control and not care any more, but severe issues of drug abuse arise, which can not only injure the patient, but also jeopardize the doctor's license. Drug abusers frequently elect not to have their condition treated. Avoiding treatment, the drug abuser may legitimately seek prescription medications from several doctors, often at the same time.

- **Withdrawing socially,** isolating oneself. This behavior is usually an overt sign of clinical depression, and must be addressed or else a downward spiral of depression ensues, disrupting the lives of the patient and his or her family members. The sufferer totally resigns himself to pain. He gives up. He might quit his job even if the pain isn't debilitating. Also, if offered part-time work, he will decline. He ceases all hobbies or activities including visiting with family and friends or going to church, choosing to suffer in silence and ignores any sympathy. He will often focus all his attention on obtaining social security or other forms of disability.

- **Blaming others** or something for the painful condition. This often occurs after treatment for the painful condition fails. In 1983, I conducted a study of 135 patients, all of whom were suffering with various types of pain syndromes. On average, I was the sixth doctor they'd seen for their complaints. Many blamed others for their painful conditions, often, former doctors. Pain managers probably most fear this kind of patient because these sufferers tend to sue.

- **Seeking direction from authoritarian** figures. Some people totally comply with the doctor, almost to the point of committing intellectual suicide. They do whatever told and abandon all thinking or questioning.

- **Blaming oneself** and living in self-pity. Like those who withdraw from society, these people are generally depressed and isolate themselves from family, friends, and life in general.

- **Blaming God** or if they have no faith, blaming fate itself. Often, these people suffer tremendous guilt and act as if destined to suffer from pain because of past sins or mistakes they've made in life.

- **Manipulating circumstances and others.** With some people, "Pain rarely occurs without an audience." In other words, some people exhibit painful behavior when around certain other people, but when alone, seem to be fine. This is not always the case and this learned behavior is usually only a problem when taken to the extreme. However, some "gain with pain" and they perceive that their pain is far more un-bearable than it physically should be. Whether actual or perceived (or both), the pain is real to the one afflicted and generally, to family members and far too often, to healthcare workers as well.

Proper Sleep

We all need sufficient and good sleep, but especially if we're suffering with any type of chronic pain. In fact, a lack of sleep is one of the major complaints of those who are caught in the vicious cycle of chronic, unrelenting pain.

There are two types of sleep. The first, rapid eye move-ment (or, REM sleep) is a period of increased activity, when we dream, when you are restless. Our heart rate, blood pres-sure, and breathing rate all increase.

The second type of sleep is termed non- rapid eye move-ment (or, NREM) sleep. During NREM sleep, our body functions and brain activity slow down. It's during the deep-est portion of NREM sleep that we experience our best, most restful sleep.

NREM sleep is divided into three stages or phases:

- Light sleep, where our body movements decrease, and we may spontaneously awaken

- Intermediate sleep, where we spend most of our sleep-ing time, refreshing our body

- Deep sleep, which is the time when it's most difficult to be aroused, and when we receive our most restor-ative sleep.

Throughout the night, we continually move from one stage of sleep to another. Deep sleep is the most restful type. Usually, we have four to six sleep cycles, each lasting 70 to 90 minutes. At the end of each cycle, we're nearly awake.

If you awaken unrested, frequently awaken, or have trouble falling back to sleep, you probably haven't reached the deep sleep stage. Do these sleep disturbances sound familiar? They should if you suffer with chronic pain because chronic pain patients can't drift into deep sleep. That's why we often prescribe certain medications to help chronic pain patients descend into deep, restful and restorative sleep (see Chapter 12).

To help you sleep better, try some of these techniques:

- Relax. Take a warm bath; practice relaxation techniques; read, write, listen to soothing music.

- Set regular sleeping hours. Go to bed and get up at the same time each day. Try to get 8 hours of sleep each night, but don't sleep-in, as this enjoyable activity tends to intensify pain.

- Avoid alcohol, caffeine and smoking, as all these are stimulants.

- Reduce interruptions. Create a low but steady background noise (e.g., a clock radio with an automatic shut-off). Keep your bedroom door closed and keep the room temperature as comfortable as possible.

- Limit activities in your bed. Use your bed for sleeping and intimacy only. Don't do work or watch a lot of TV in bed.

- Establish a regular work-out time each day, but earlier in the day, as physical activity causes a release of certain chemicals in your body which may stimulate, not sedate you.

- Don't try to sleep. Read or listen to the radio until you become drowsy. If you can't get to sleep, get up and do some work around the house. Gradually, you'll feel sleepy.

- If you nap during the day, sleep no longer than 30 minutes, and take your nap in the mid-afternoon.

If you still have problems sleeping, talk with your doctor. There are many supplements, herbs, and prescription medications which can help you sleep better.

Depression

Many chronic pain sufferers develop another complex and frustrating illness: depression. This component of chronic pain is often termed suffering. The term depression refers to a sad mood or emotion that may be a normal reaction to an important unhappy life event such as divorce, death of a loved one, or a business failure.

Depression may not be the accurate diagnosis of one suffering chronically with pain. The term may more appropriately be termed a *depressed mood*. A depressed mood implies that the patient exhibits depressed symptoms at times, but at other times, he or she is not depressed. To me, this makes more sense than a specific diagnosis of depression, because for one to be truly diagnosed with depression, the patient must experience in the same two weeks, five or more of the following symptoms:

- A depressed mood. For most of nearly every day, the patient reports a depressed mood.

- A marked decrease in interests or pleasure.

- A marked loss or gain of weight or a marked decrease or increase in appetite.

- Unusual sleep patterns. Nearly every day the patient sleeps excessively or not enough.

- Changes in the patient's activities, either slowed or speeded up.

- Tiredness or loss of energy.

- Feeling worthless or inappropriately guilty.

- Indecisiveness or inability to concentrate.

- Repeated thoughts of suicide.

With chronic pain, depression may be a normal development but yet, distinctly different from the pain itself. Depression actually refers to a group of several distinct psychiatric syndromes characterized by long periods of constant, severe, and extensive mood changes. Initially, this depression is caused by an increase in production of some of the chemicals made in the brain (neurotransmitters). These chemicals produce personality changes and prevent the sufferer from obtaining a good night's sleep. In fact, the chronic pain patient develops an unconscious addiction to these, his very own neurotransmitters and depends upon the personality changes that develop.

In addition to sleep disturbances, depression from chronic pain also affects work performance, sexual drive, and all other emotions. Depressed people feel worthless, tired, unforgivable; rise early in the morning, think slowly, and may think thoughts of suicide. Depression often leads to over-eating and weight gain, both of which only serve to intensify the depression.

Depression also often arises from undiagnosed pain. Most are told that the pain is "All in their heads." Have you heard that before? This is especially true of those involved in motor vehicle accidents who have been forced to file suit against insurance companies to have their medical bills and lost wages paid. They are accused of faking the pain and malingering. Sadly, many doctors themselves don't believe these patients and frequently convince family members also that there is no cause for such pain. Do you think these folks developed depression? Absolutely!

Unfortunately, depressed people tend to blame everyone, including doctors, clinics, or therapists, for their loss of control over their lives and altered life style. They frequently "doctor shop", and when disappointed, then "attorney shop" to sue former doctors.

Chapter Summary

Pain is a private experience, but pain behavior is governed by our social and cultural backgrounds. We can only observe one's behavior as he or she expresses a perception of pain. Pain is usually a misused word in social discourse when we are actually referring to suffering.

Pain's complexities remind me of our human complexities, the idea expressed in David's Psalm 139, "You are fearfully and wonderfully made."

Each of us interprets the sensation of pain in different manners at different times in our lives. Generally, we exhibit reaction to pain based upon many psychological factors. Many change as we age; yet some, like cultural or ethnic influences, seem to remain throughout our lifetime.

Doctors who treat patients suffering with painful disorders must incorporate the psychological and spiritual facets as well as the physical. It's both foolish and arrogant for a doctor to ignore the fact that we truly, are "fearfully and wonderfully made."

References

1. **Swanson DW (ed).** *Mayo Clinic on Chronic Pain.* Rochester: Mayo Clinic, 1999.

2. **Oates WE, Oates CE.** *People in Pain: Guidelines for Pastoral Care.* Philadelphia: Westminster Press, 1985.

3. **Marcus NJ.** *Freedom from Chronic Pain.* New York: Simon & Schuster, 1994.

4. **Morrison J.** *DSM-IV Made Easy: The Clinician's Guide to Diagnosis.* New York: The Guilford Press;1995:190-194.

CHAPTER Three

Trigeminal Neuralgia

Neuralgia and neuritis are often confused and improperly used to mean nerve pain. Webster defines neuralgia as, "Pain along a nerve." If you suffer with any nerve pain, this phrase may seem accurate. Actually, it's only partially correct.

Neuritis refers to an inflammatory process associated with a nerve or root of a nerve (for example, as the nerve comes off the spinal cord). Inflammation produces a constant, burning pain and if the source of the inflammation is treatable, neuritis is curable.

By contrast, neuralgia often has no known pathological cause . . . nor can one be found, except in rare occasions. Exceptions exist, but usually causes for neuralgia escape us. The pain is highly intense and episodic. If the source of neuralgia can't be found, doctors are frustrated and patients are desperate. Such desperation, unfortunately, often leads to inappropriate, invasive, and destructive treatment.

Consider neuralgia as pain with a nerve and its connections to the central nervous system. That doesn't necessarily mean that neuralgias don't occur outside the central nervous system (for example, in a tooth or bone), but often, neuralgia pain is felt to be outside the central nervous system when the problem actually originates inside the brain.

A terrible disorder of the trigeminal or fifth cranial nerve, trigeminal neuralgia, is probably the most excruciating type of pain plaguing mankind. As many as 1.6 million people in the United States alone are afflicted with trigeminal neuralgia.

Such is the case with trigeminal neuralgia. From the beginning of recorded history, healers and sufferers alike have frantically searched for a cure of this dreaded disease which, although not life-threatening, has driven many to the brink of suicide . . . and beyond.

A terrible disorder of the trigeminal or fifth cranial nerve, trigeminal neuralgia, is probably the most excruciating type of pain plaguing mankind. As many as 1.6 million people in the United States alone are afflicted with trigeminal neuralgia.

History of Trigeminal Neuralgia

In the first century A.D., Aretaeus described a painful condition of the face and head, which some medical historians have interpreted as trigeminal neuralgia (TGN). The earliest recorded description of actual trigeminal neuralgia is that of the eleventh century Arab physician Jurani.

In 1688, a description of TGN was actually published as a eulogy to Johannes Baush, who apparently during the end of his life suffered from severe facial pain, prohibiting him from speaking or chewing.

Nicholas Andre published the first scientific description of TGN in 1756. He coined the French and common name, *tic douloureux*, which literally means *unbearably painful twitch*.

Seventeen years later, John Fothergill described 14 cases of trigeminal neuralgia in such detail that the disease became known as Fothergill's disease. His descriptions are still accurate today.

John Locke wrote the first complete description of trigeminal neuralgia in 1677. Locke (1632-1704), a physician, political scientist, and philosopher, was asked to examine the wife of the English ambassador to France, the Countess of Northumberland. After his examination, he wrote detailed descriptions of his findings to four physicians in England, asking for their advice.

Dr. John Mecklethwaite, President of the Royal College of Physicians, replied to Locke, stating: "But because the pain is most urgent it will be necessary to give opiates inwardly and apply little sponges or linens dipped in syrup of castor and liquid landanum to the part pained and apply large blisters under the ear and under the armpit of the side effected."

Sir Charles Scarburgh wrote Locke and recommended, " . . . leaches to the gum itself or cauterizing the gum to the very bottom." Understand that local anesthetic wasn't invented until nearly 1900, so one would have to really be suffering to undergo cauterization or burning of the tissue with a red hot instrument without an anesthetic!

As early as the late 17th century, treatment for trigeminal neuralgia branched into two directions, as in all medicine: use of medicine and surgery. This diversity continues even today. Some doctors list, under their names, "Physician and Surgeon" This tradition originated in the late 17th century.

From the beginning, treatment of trigeminal neuralgia has been barbaric and only slightly effective at best. Historically, some of the types of treatment used have been: the application of tar (1814), steam (1839) and ice (1873) to the face; carotid artery ligation (1862); local galvanic stimulation of the nerve (1870); vibration to the face (1884); radiotherapy (1897); adjustment of the dental occlusion (1912); diathermy (1916); appendectomy (1916); removal of styloid process (1921); mastoidectomy (1927); sectioning of the great auricular nerve (1953) and of the greater occipital nerve (1954); injection of hot water (1959), phenol in glycerin (1963) and glycerol (1981) directly into the trigeminal ganglion; and crushing portions of the trigeminal ganglion with a balloon (1983).

As recently as 1930, plunging the opposite hand into boiling water was advocated to relieve the horrible pain of TGN. This treatment alone demonstrates the desperation with which some patients sought relief.

In my practice, I see many of these unfortunate sufferers. Believe me, most will do anything to gain just a few moments of relief from their torment. Some come disfigured and maimed. Others simply come with the hope of finding even slight relief. TGN is the most challenging of all the craniofacial pain syndromes we encounter. Even partial relief of the torment of pain is reward enough.

Different Types of Trigeminal Neuralgia

Trigeminal neuralgia can be divided into three distinct disorders:

1. Typical trigeminal neuralgia;

2. Atypical trigeminal neuralgia; and

3. Atypical facial pain.

Doctors frequently confuse these three, for most don't even know separate categories exist. Far too often, when a person suffers severe facial pain with no apparent cause, the diagnosis is trigeminal neuralgia, but which of the three is correct? Proper treatment depends on the doctor discovering an accurate diagnosis. Sadly, many of you reading this will know more about the various types of trigeminal neuralgia than most doctors.

Typical Trigeminal Neuralgia

Typical trigeminal neuralgia (TTN), classically known as tic douloureux, usually afflicts persons in their fifties or older. Compression of the trigeminal nerve in the skull by a tiny blood vessel appears to be the main cause. Approximately 6% of TTN sufferers also have multiple sclerosis, so often, multiple sclerosis is the actual diagnosis, TTN being the secondary problem.

The symptoms of tic douloureux are obvious: sharp electrical pain, which lasts for seconds (Table 3.1). Washing, shaving, applying makeup, brushing the teeth, kissing, or even cold air blowing over the specific area triggers the pain. The second division of the trigeminal nerve (the maxillary division), which supplies feeling to the mid-face, upper teeth and palate, seems to be most involved. The pain is so severe that the sufferer will do virtually anything to avoid touching the trigger zone.

I teach students, residents and colleagues to inject a local anesthetic to numb the affected trigeminal nerve branch to discover which portion may be causing the neuralgia. If the local anesthetic injection doesn't stop ALL the pain, then either something else is wrong or the problem may stem from inside the skull where the trigeminal nerve comes off the brain.

We treat TTN with medications (medications are discussed in much more detail in Chapter 12). Historically, Tegretal has been the drug of choice for orofacial pain, especially TTN. It's effective, but the side effects (fatigue, drowsiness, damage to blood marrow cells) often discourage patients from taking Tegretal for any length of time.

Baclofen is a more recent drug. Its side effects (fatigue, dry mouth, and drowsiness) don't seem as severe and if the doctor gradually increases the dosage, these side effects are generally overcome.

A third and newer medication, Neurontin, has been miraculous in its benefits. The side effects are similar to those of Tegretal and Baclofen, and again, the dosage can be slowly increased to avoid severe side effects.

We also prescribe Dilantin and Klonopin, two common drugs used to treat epilepsy, in combination with Tegretal. These combinations are very effective, but unfortunately, cause drowsiness. Klonopin, for TNN, is often given at bedtime.

If treatment with medications is unsuccessful, then we treat the individual branches of the trigeminal nerve with local anesthetic and cortisone injections, but rarely is this successful with typical trigeminal neuralgia. I've had some success with these injections when used together with one or several of the drugs mentioned above.

Some neurosurgeons inject alcohol or glycerin directly into sections of the nerve (called a neurolytic block) to purposely damage the fibers of the nerve, which carry pain sensations. Usually, this produces a long-lasting anesthesia. Unfortunately, I've not had much success with his type of injection. It's difficult to limit damage to surrounding structures and often, we must repeat this painful procedure.

If all else fails, we consider brain surgery. This decision would be made with a neurosurgeon, who has several different surgical procedures to consider. The most common and successful (at least for my patients) is termed microvascular decompression. Dr. Peter Jennetta devised this very intricate procedure while he was still a neurosurgery resident. When my patients require this procedure, they're referred to Dr. Jennetta in Pittsburgh.

Another successful brain surgery procedure for typical trigeminal neuralgia is named percutaneous radio frequency thermoneurolysis. For this procedure, the neurosurgeon places an electrode directly into the Gasserian ganglion (the trigeminal ganglion) and with radio waves, actually cauterizes and destroys sections of the main divisions of the trigeminal nerve. Obviously, this destructive procedure may produce undesirable side effects such as muscle paralysis, dry eyes, and at times, an increase in pain.

Balloon rhizotomy or balloon decompression procedure, which is similar to balloon angioplasty for opening clogged vessels in the heart, is another surgical option. The neurosurgeon inserts a small fiber through the skin in the cheek into the trigeminal or gasserian ganglion. A small balloon at the end is then inflated, causing slight damage to the nerve by placing pressure on the nerve fibers, injuring them so that pain impulses can no longer be passed on.

Another procedure, which is non-invasive, is termed stereotactic radiosurgery, or gamma knife. The patient's head is held in place with a custom head-holder, which has 201 strategically placed holes. A lesion is created on the trigeminal nerve root by delivering a single highly concentrated dose of ionizing radiation through the 201 holes, to a small, precise target at the point of pain origination. There's minimum exposure to healthy surrounding brain tissue. Because gamma knife radiosurgery is non-invasive, we avoid many complications likely with open brain surgery, and it requires only a one-night hospitalization. Loss of feeling in the face is rare with gamma knife treatment.

All surgical procedures have inherent risks. If you or a loved one is considering surgery for trigeminal neuralgia, seek a second or third opinion. Ask the neurosurgeon about these surgical techniques and why he or she is recommending a specific type of surgery. Remember to ask the surgeon about possible post-operative complications as well as his or hers experience and success rate. You might even ask to speak with a patient or two who've undergone the recommended surgery.

If you or a loved one is considering surgery for trigeminal neuralgia, seek a second or third opinion.

Atypical Trigeminal Neuralgia

In contrast to the typical kind, atypical trigeminal neuralgia (ATN) causes pain constantly with the intensity increasing and decreasing, almost like crescendos and decescendos of a symphony. Atypical trigeminal neuralgia also has trigger zones; however, there's also an area of dull aching, which is intensified by touching the trigger zones, often causing shooting pains. These shooting pains, which resemble tic douloureux, often confuse both patient and doctor.

The patient is often diagnosed with the typical type of trigeminal neuralgia (Table 3.1). In my clinical experience, this is the most common type of trigeminal neu-

> *Atypical trigeminal neuralgia is the most common type of trigeminal neuralgia.*

ralgia. It's so common, that rarely a week passes without one or two new patients being diagnosed with ATN in my office.

According to the medical literature, ATN affects all three divisions of the trigeminal nerve equally. However, in my practice, I don't see this equal distribution of facial pain. Rather, the most common areas I see are below the eye (the infraorbital nerve) and the middle of the lower jaw (the mental nerve).

A common cause of this disorder is trauma, especially after a surgical incision (for example, the surgical removal of a tooth or the placement of a dental implant), a root canal, or a blow to the face.

It's important to rule-out other problems in order to establish a diagnosis of atypical trigeminal neuralgia (for example, an abscessed tooth or sinus infection). The trigeminal nerve branch, which is producing pain, is injected with a local anesthetic to eliminate the pain. This is like turning off various circuits in a circuit breaker box to see which electrical circuit powers the dishwasher, for example.

We treat atypical trigeminal neuralgia by injecting an anti-inflammatory medication into the injured nerve branch area and prescribing Baclofen or Neurontin. Sometimes we prescribe oral synthetic cortisone like your physician may prescribe for you after a bee sting (usually called a dosepak). Often we have to repeat the injections several times, but we're successful in eliminating the terrible neuralgia symptoms about 65% to 70% of the time.

We've also had great success treating ATN with a combination of injections and oral medications, such as Baclofen or Neurontin. Many of our patients get to the point where they require injections only once every 12 to 24 months, as long as they take their oral medication daily.

If this conservative therapy is not successful, then we consider surgery, which may involve the injection of alcohol or glycerol to destroy the nerve. Some pain doctors use a freezing procedure termed cryoanalgesia, which freezes the nerve with liquid nitrogen, destroying the pain-carrying fibers.

I use percutaneous radio frequency thermoneurolysis to treat ATN surgically. After the offending trigeminal nerve branch is numbed with a local anesthetic injection, I place a special electrode near, on, or in the nerve. Satisfied that I have the proper placement of the electrode, I instruct my surgical assistant to turn the radio frequency generator on, which creates energy to destroy the portions of the trigeminal nerve, which convey pain sensations. Usually, the portions of the nerve, which carry pressure or temperature sensations, aren't injured. Sometimes they are, but generally they heal within a few weeks to a few months.

As with all surgical procedures, there are risks with radio frequency thermoneurolysis. Rarely, few patients see no improvement. Other possible, but rare side effects are anesthesia dolorosa (numbness with increased, constant, burning pain), only partial relief, and possible injury to other nerves. ATN patients feel that any amount of relief of pain is worth these risks.

We have to re-treat about 17% to 20% of the surgical cases within 5 years because the nervous system attempts to repair the injury caused by the radio frequency procedure. Like all destructive procedures used to reduce or eliminate pain, success may be reduction but not total elimination of the pain. You and your doctor have to decide what constitutes acceptable success. In my years of clinical experience, I can't recall a patient suffering from atypical trigeminal neuralgia who was upset if most, but not all the pain was relieved.

Atypical Facial Pain

Atypical facial pain (AFP) is a disorder that also affects the trigeminal nerve However, the symptoms are not clearly defined as they are in the typical and atypical types (Table 3.1).

Atypical facial pain is usually continuous with no triggers. Proper identification of the cause of this type of trigeminal pain is not very successful. Therefore, those suffering with AFP are most often mistreated and ill-treated. Unfortunately, by the time I see these poor folks, they've usually had multiple root canals with subsequent removal of the teeth. Some have had several neurosurgeries, and most are dependent upon strong prescription medications.

Proper identification of the cause of this type of trigeminal pain is not very successful. Therefore, those suffering with AFP are most often mistreated and ill-treated.

Atypical facial pain seems to afflict people who are under a tremendous amount of stress and many seem to have a history of psychiatric problems. This doesn't mean that people with AFP are mentally ill, just that no absolute, diagnostic test for atypical facial pain exits. Many symptoms and types of patients are thrown into this nebulous category. That isn't fair or accurate.

In my practice, I've not found but two or three patients with this problem who also needed psychological counseling and then, I had to wonder if that was because no one believed their complaints of facial pain. Also, as with most of us in today's fast-paced society, stress is a major factor in our lives.

Those with AFP do seem to be affected more by stress. When doctors can't find the immediate cause for a pain disorder and the patient suffers from stress (who doesn't?), then it's assumed that a psychological cause explains the undiagnosed pain.

In contrast to the effects of stress, some atypical facial pain problems seem to be caused by psychological problems. These are generally the patients who have constant, deep and

Table 3.1: Comparisons of trigeminal neuralgia (typical and atypical) and atypical facial pain.			
Pain	**Typical TGN**	**Atypical TGN**	**Atypical Facial Pain**
Character	Sharp	Dull	Varies
Duration	Seconds	Constant	Constant
Frequency	Intermittent	Constant	Constant
Location	V2* & V3+	All 3 Divisions	Vague
Triggers	Extra-Oral	Varies	Vague
Stress Induced	No	No	Possibly
V2*: Maxillary division of the trigeminal nerve			
V3+: Mandibular division of the trigeminal nerve			

dull pain, which may last days, months or even years. Facial movements, activities or contact don't effect the pain, but fatigue, stress, worry, and general emotional turmoil aggravate the pain. These people also experience pain that often crosses the midline of the face and affects both sides of the face, and that type of pain is considered psychogenic pain (pain that's not caused by damaged or perceived damaged tissue).

Sufferers of AFP tend to over-dramatize their symptoms in what I can only describe as a bizarre or very exaggerated manner. For example, in addition to reported facial pain, the patient may complain of difficulty with swallowing and a feeling of heaviness of his cheeks lying against his upper teeth.

Augmentation, a variation of atypical facial pain that Mumford, an English orofacial pain researcher described, produces ATP. Sufferers are more aware of their face and mouth than usual. This condition frustrates the dentist who, after placing a perfectly good restoration (i.e., dental filling), finds the patient continually complaining of shooting or sharp pains in the face or mouth. This isn't too unusual because we all know people who can't stand to wear tight clothing, watchbands, or jewelry. The reticular activating system, a brain section, was created to alert us of such stimuli, is overly activated. Probably one or two of these augmenting patients appear in my office per month.

A similar irritation is the ticking of a clock when you're trying to study. You know what I mean. Until you engross yourself in your reading or studies, every tick is distracting and at times, you want to scream.

Patients with mouth augmentation give dentists nightmares. After having occlusion (i.e., bite) adjusted by the dentist, the patient develops a type of augmentation called occlusal awareness disease. Not actually a disease per se, this psychogenic abnormal awareness of one's teeth contacting may lead to atypical facial pain, yet the actual cause is rarely discovered.

For those with atypical facial pain, it's so important for the sufferer to have patience with the doctor or doctors and for those frustrated clinicians to have patience with the sufferer. Often, out of desperation on everyone's part, invasive and irreparable procedures are conducted in an attempt to, quite honestly, quiet and appease the patient. This is very unfortunate and only makes matters worse.

Generally, if we assure the patient with AFP that his or her complaints are not a result of cancer or some other dreaded disease, the patient's demanding behavior is lessoned. I find that taking time and listening to the patient's complaints with genuine interest goes a long way toward reducing his or her AFP symptoms. If the doctor listens and spends time with the patient, trust and mutual respect are formed, and unnecessary destructive procedures can be avoided.

If you or a loved one suffers with atypical facial pain, please don't try to force the doctor's hands concerning your treatment. When I think back over the past 23 years or so of my practice, I'm not proud to confess I've made more errors of judgement with AFP patients than any other category of patients. Learn from my mistakes.

Treatment for atypical facial pain must be directed towards elimination of the symptoms. Medications, anesthetic injections and stress management are helpful . . . at times. Avoid surgery unless a specific structure producing pain symptoms can be isolated. Perhaps the torment of neuralgia may best be described in the poem "Faith, Hope and Love", (on page 56) written by one who suffers daily with pain.

"Faith, Hope and Love"

There is a Beast Amongst me
It lingers all day long
No matter what I do or take,
This Beast is never gone.

No one sees this Ghastly Beast
No, not even I.
But, I know it is in there,
"Please God, Don't let me Die."

I have traveled many roads
Hoping to find a cure.
Doctors, Dentists have no clue,
Of what I have endured.

No plans dare I make,
As it may upset this Beast.
I now take tiny Baby Steps,
To say the very least.

I must not look back
On that fatal dental day.
For I know I must move forward
And hear what others have to say.

For those out there, like me,
I pray each and every night,
Asking God to lend His Hand,
And listen to our plight.

There are many of us suffering,
This I truly know.
But, Miracles can happen
With the "Hope and Love"
we show.

Written by
Mary R. Whitney ©1999.

~ ~ ~ ~ ~ ~
This is dedicated to all those
suffering in pain,
especially to
Facial Neuralgic Victims.
~ ~ ~ ~ ~ ~

Chapter Summary ——

Trigeminal neuralgia is a debilitating disease, which is not fatal, but produces some of the most intense pain one may suffer. There are three separate types, but many doctors lump all three into one category termed tic douloureux.

The more common type, atypical trigeminal neuralgia, responds well to medical treatment about 70% of the time.

Atypical facial pain is a composite of facial pain and psychological symptoms. This type of trigeminal nerve pain drives many patients and doctors to attempt almost any type of therapy. Unfortunately, many patients receive improper and damaging treatment, often leading to doctor shopping and medication abuse.

An accurate diagnosis must be established before any invasive procedures are considered. Patients have the right to know the source of their pain before they submit to any type of treatment. Ask the doctor to explain in detail the type of therapy that he or she recommends. Remember to discuss possible side effects and alternative treatments.

CHAPTER Four

Odontalgia

A book written about facial pain must include a chapter on tooth pain, or odontalgia. Simple as it may seem, it's often hard to diagnosis properly the cause of a toothache. Many factors affect pain sensitivity of teeth. Sometimes the cause is straightforward: a large cavity. Other times, diagnosis eludes the dentist, to the annoyance of the sufferer.

Nerves in Those Teeth

Inside each healthy tooth is a complex conglomeration of tissues collectively termed the pulp, which is composed of blood vessels, nerves, and lymphatic tissue. In a sense, each pulp is an organ with the ability to sense pain, changes in temperature, pressure, and chemical irritants. For upper teeth, the nerves are branches of the maxillary division of the trigeminal nerve. Lower teeth nerves are branches of the mandibular division of the trigeminal nerve. Some lower teeth also have branches of cervical nerves, which is one reason why your dentist may have trouble numbing your lower back teeth.

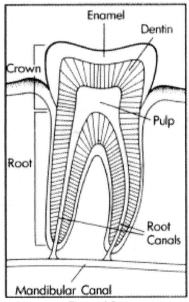

Figure 4.1:
Drawing of tooth anatomy.

Nerve fibers enter the tooth through an opening near the tip of the root (the apical foramen) and travel through the pulp as several large bundles in a fairly straight course towards the pulp chamber within the crown (Figure 4.1). Arriving in the pulp chamber, the nerves then divide and travel to cells called odontoblasts, cells comprising the layer of the tooth termed the dentin. The dentin is the darker, more organic layer below the enamel of the crown.

The crown of the tooth is non-living. Once formed in the jawbone, the enamel receives neither nourishment nor blood and is incapable of sensation. Only after enamel is fractured or decayed (forming a cavity or cavitation in the enamel) can the underlying dentin perceive sensations, especially pain. Enamel is as hard as diamond, but over years, it wears and can fracture.

The outside surface of the roots of teeth receive their nerve supply from minute branches of the trigeminal nerve, which are separate branches from the nerves inside the tooth. That's why you can still sense tooth pain at times even after the inside nerve has been removed by your dentist (a root canal procedure).

Dental Decay

Dental decay, or caries, is one of the most common diseases known to mankind. Several different microorganisms, unique to the mouth, produce acid in the presence of sugar. Over time, the acid breaks through the enamel, forming a cavity (or carious lesion), exposing the dentin. It takes a long time to form a cavity, but once one develops, the underlying organic dentin is exposed. That's when you feel pain or at least sensitivity.

If you have a cavity, often you don't feel pain until food or liquids are trapped within the cavity, stimulating pain fibers in the dentin. The tooth can be sensitive to cold temperatures, sugar, or breathing in cold air.

Due to the pain's intensity and pain radiation, isolating the specific tooth is often difficult for both patient and dentist.

Initially, toothache pain from a cavity is generalized and you may have a difficulty pointing to the specific tooth. That's why your dentist or dental hygienist takes bitewing x-rays, or x-ray films which show between the teeth. Pulpal pain lasts a long time and is excruciating. Due to the pain's intensity and pain radiation, isolating the specific tooth is often difficult for both patient and dentist.

Trying to find an infected tooth, we sometimes use an electronic pulp tester on several teeth in the area. This small, battery operated device, produces a small tingling sensation when a healthy tooth is touched. We also apply ice to test teeth. If a tooth has a cavity, ice intensifies the pain. If abscessed, ice reduces the tooth's pain.

Without dental repair, a tooth will continue to decay until the advancing cavity contacts the pulp. Inflammation forms, which is followed by infection. An abscess quickly forms as the pulpal tissue within the tooth dies and disintegrates (Figure 4.2).

A tooth abscess causes an infection in the bone which contains the tooth. Swelling develops, the tooth seems higher than all the other teeth, and what was once a mild or moderate painful irritation becomes an intense, painful condition. Often, a fever develops, and temperatures, especially warmth, make the pain worse.

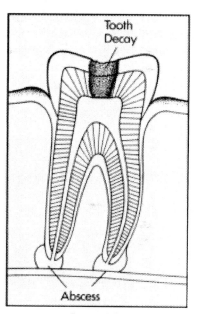

Figure 4.2:
Abscessed tooth.

If an abscess forms, you may feel tired and generally sick. Your lymph nodes swell and you may develop an earache. Others symptoms may include bad breath and a foul taste in your mouth.

A tooth developing an abscess won't always show on an x-ray. This makes diagnosis difficult for the doctor, as he may think the problem is trauma from occlusion, or biting too hard on that tooth. Sometimes it takes a week or more before an abscess is evident on the x-ray film. I frequently see patients who've been referred by excellent doctors only to discover an abscess when I perform an examination. Finding an abscess makes me look good, but I make sure the patient understands that the referring doctor was handicapped in his evaluation because the initial abscess wasn't visible on the x-ray.

Abscessed teeth can seriously threaten your health. Before the advent of antibiotics, people died from these localized diseases. Dental caries are still life-threatening in third-world countries, and that's why many missionary doctors are dentists. It's not hard to understand that you can't share the Gospel with someone if he or she has a severe toothache. To paraphrase Thomas Aquinas, "Stop a man's toothache pain and then tell him about Christ."

Today, we treat abscessed teeth one of two ways: remove the offending tooth or treat the disease with a minor surgical procedure termed root canal therapy. If the abscess isn't treated quickly, we may have to make an incision in the gum tissues and at times, a hole in the bone, to allow the abscess to drain before providing any other therapy. In such severe cases, we also prescribe an antibiotic.

Discuss your options with your dentist. Today there's great controversy concerning root canal therapy (see Chapter 7). Millions of teeth have been saved by endodontic (root canal) techniques, but, there's mounting evidence that for some patients, it may be better to remove dead or dying teeth instead of attempting to save them with root canal therapy. Extraction or root canal therapy is your choice. Remember, doctors work for you, including your dentist. If you're not satisfied with your dentist's explanations, get a second opinion.

For the most part, we can prevent dental caries and tooth abscesses with good oral hygiene and regular visits to the dentist. At times, teeth die and abscesses form for no known reason, but this is rare. Seeing your dentist on a regular basis will allow the doctor to detect any problems before they become severe.

If you experience any of the following symptoms, see your dentist as soon as possible:

- Tooth sensitivity to temperatures or when chewing
- Continuous or throbbing tooth pain
- Fever when there's no other obvious reason (the flu, for example)
- Earache when your physician can't find a cause
- Neck or jaw tenderness or swollen glands on the same side as the toothache
- General ill feeling when your physician can't find any cause
- Bad breath or a foul taste in your mouth

What can you do for yourself until you see your dentist? To reduce pain and fever, take over-the-counter medications like aspirin or ibuprofen. Acetaminophen will reduce pain but not fever. Never place a crushed aspirin on the painful tooth or gum tissues beside the tooth. You'll seriously burn the soft tissues of your mouth and from such a burn, you can cause a ripe environment for other types of infections to develop.

If you have swelling, apply ice to the side of your face. Avoid drinking extremely cold or hot liquids. If hot temperatures increase your pain, be assured you have an abscess. If you're only bothered with cold temperatures, you probably have a deep cavity.

Avoid sweets and hot, spicy foods. You might have to stick to a luke-warm liquid diet until you can see your dentist.

Lastly, rinse your mouth with warm salt water or mouthwash to reduce the bacteria in your mouth. Once an abscess forms, other bacteria will grow quickly, and rinsing with these solutions will prevent additional mouth infections.

Probably the best advice I can give you is to see your dentist if you have any tooth sensitivity. Often, we can easily (and painlessly, believe it or not!) treat cavities which are early in their development. Avoiding the dentist is not a good idea.

Cracked Tooth Syndrome

Today, people are keeping their teeth longer (for life, we hope) thanks to advances in dental procedures and routine visits to the dentist. Any tooth may crack, especially one which already has a cavity or a large restoration (filling). Exposing teeth to years of eating hard foods, chewing ice, or grinding increases the chances that the enamel in one or several will crack.

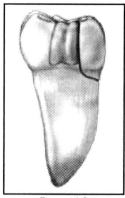

**Figure 4.3:
Fractured cusp.**

If a corner of enamel fractures, the only pain you'll experience sometimes is temperature sensitivity or roughness to your tongue. We treat that problem by simply restoring the fractured tooth, usually with a crown (cap) or gold onlay, if one of the cusps are fractured (Figure 4.3).

Other times, minute cracks occur, producing intermittent pain when chewing, especially between bites as you release the pressure on the fractured tooth (Figure 4.4). You may also feel pain when eating or drinking something hot or cold. This type of crack makes it very difficult for you to isolate the cracked tooth because the pain comes and goes. And if you think it's hard for you to find the cracked tooth, its even more difficult for your dentist. You may have to return to the dentist's office several times before the doctor finally discovers the offending tooth, if he or she ever does.

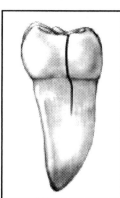

**Figure 4.4:
Cracked tooth
(vertical fracture).**

Cracked teeth rarely show up on x-rays. If we're fortunate, taking x-rays from two or three different directions sometimes helps, but this is rare. We also apply a dye (methylene blue) to teeth to show us where the crack is located, but this diagnostic procedure is difficult to perform because of saliva. Your dentist might shine a bright light (translumination) directed at different angles trying to detect fracture lines.

If you have a cracked tooth, you may, unconsciously, begin to chew on the opposite only. Generally, we chew mostly on our dominate side: if we're right handed, we'll chew on the right side more than the left. If you don't believe this, look in the mirror and see which side of your face is just a little bit larger. You'll see it's your dominate side. So, if you crack a tooth on your dominate side, you'll start chewing on the other side, and this may cause muscle pain, especially in the temporalis and masseter muscles.

Sometimes we tap various teeth to cause the pain. Also, we may ask the patient to bite down on an instrument, trying to find the pain. From these simple diagnostic tests, we improve our chances to find a cracked tooth, if that's the pain problem.

We also often use diagnostic anesthetic injections to find the specific cracked tooth. One by one, using a technique called periodontal ligament infiltration, each tooth's nerve supply is chemically turned-off. If there's an offending tooth in the area, this test is highly successful in locating that tooth.

Why do cracked teeth hurt? That's a good question because enamel isn't living. A crack in a tooth usually affects the underlying dentin and even the pulp, stimulating nerves. If you don't apply pressure on the tooth by chewing or grinding your teeth, the fractured area of the dentin isn't stimulated.

If we discover the cracked tooth before an abscess forms, restoring the tooth (placing a filling or a crown) is all that's needed to treat the problem. Untreated cracked teeth often split, making them nearly impossible to save.

How can you prevent your teeth from cracking? Cracked teeth can't be completely prevented, but there are steps you can take to make your teeth less susceptible to cracks:

- Don't chew on hard objects like ice, unpopped popcorn kernels, pencils or pens

- Try not to grind or clench your teeth

- If you do clench or grind your teeth, consult your dentist about getting an appliance to protect your teeth

- Always wear a protective mouth guard when playing contact sports

- If you experience symptoms of a cracked tooth, see your dentist as soon as possible

- If you're struck in the mouth in a fight or in an accident, see your dentist

- Place a piece of wax (available at drug stores) over the cracked area (if possible) until you see your dentist

One final comment about tooth fractures: As an Ohio State graduate (multiple times!), a former member of the best marching band in the land, and an avid football fan, I admired Coach Woody Hayes. In the 1950s and 60s, Ohio State football was known as, "three yards and a cloud of dust." In those years, Woody rarely allowed his quarterbacks to pass the football because, as the Coach would say, "Three things can happen when you pass the ball, and two of them are bad." Sometimes when fixing large decayed areas in teeth, we have to place tiny pins in the tooth to hold the filling material. Just like passing the football, three things can happen every time a dentist places a pin in a tooth, and two of them are bad: (1) the pin may inadvertently go into the pulp of the tooth, (2) the tooth may fracture; or (3) the pin may be properly secured in the tooth, causing no damage. Sometimes, the fracture isn't noticed for weeks.

If your dentist places a pin or two in your tooth, just think of Coach Hayes . . . no, just kidding. Realize you may develop an iatrogenic (a bad result as a result of good medical care) fracture. If you develop cracked tooth symptoms, go back to your dentist immediately.

Temperature Sensitivity

Many of us experience tooth sensitivity due to cold temperatures. Dental decay isn't the only cause of this type of sensitivity.

If you have gingival (gum) recession, the root surface of teeth are exposed. Root surfaces are covered with a very thin layer of cementum which, when exposed, is extremely sensitive. Sweets, acidic foods (citric fruits, tomatoes), cold temperatures, and tooth brushing all stimulate the nerves of the cementum, producing pain. This condition affects us middle-aged and older people, but if you've had orthodontic treatment or grind your teeth, you may also develop this type of pain.

Use one of the desensitizing tooth pastes available from the drug store (e.g., Sensodyne). This type of treatment may take up to six weeks or so before you see any improvement. If the temperature sensitivity continues, see your dental hygienist or dentist, as they have special medicines and sealants which, when applied to the root surfaces of the teeth, generally cure the problem. Your dentist may have to apply one of these substances every few months or years.

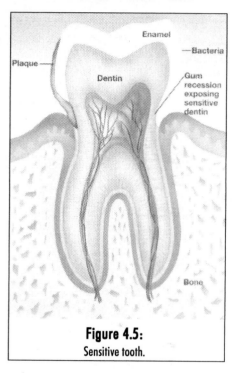

Figure 4.5:
Sensitive tooth.

I often make custom mouth guards and prescribe concentrated fluoride gel. Then I instruct my patient to wear the gel-filled mouth guards daily for about 10 minutes, usually while showering because the fluoride will make you salivate a lot. This procedure is very effective when the others fail.

Inflamed gums also cause temperature sensitivity. As plaque accumulates around the necks of your teeth, an acidic environment develops and any cold temperatures amplify the effects of this acidic environment. Have your teeth cleaned by your dental hygienist and maintain good oral hygiene habits (brushing and flossing). Use a soft, polished bristle tooth brush (Figure 4.5).

Root surfaces are covered with a very thin layer of cementum which, when exposed, is extremely sensitive.

Obviously, avoid cold and acidic foods and drinks, including carbonated drinks. Also, refrain from eating sticky foods like candy, honey, or syrup, as these tend to stick to the root surfaces of teeth.

If you use smokeless tobacco, use this as an opportunity to stop. Smokeless tobacco is not only a source of oral cancer, it also adheres to the root surfaces of teeth, causing the gingivae to recede.

If your sensitivity is caused by grinding or clenching your teeth, ask your dentist to make a mouth guard, and wear it whenever you sleep. When awake, try not to clench your teeth. Clenching during the day is usually a habit or a response to stress, so think about checking to see if you're clenching. If you are, stop. If you can't stop clenching, wear your mouth guard whenever possible.

Tooth Sensitivity After Dental Procedures

If I could solve this problem, I'd retire a rich man! Whenever we place any type of dental restoration (for example, a filling or crown), the pulp of the tooth is traumatized. You don't feel the trauma when it occurs because your dentist has numbed the tooth with a local anesthetic. In additional to the pulpal injury from a cavity or cracked tooth, the mechanical activity of the dental hand piece (or drill) produces pulpal trauma. That's why your dentist's hand piece sprays water on the tooth while drilling: The water cools the tooth, preventing the pulp from over-heating. Today's dental hand pieces are vastly improved over the ones used as recently as the 1960s, but still, the tooth must be cooled when the doctor's operating.

Dentists often place a material called a base before placing the final filling in order to protect the pulpal tissue, the tooth will still be sensitive to cold temperatures. In fact, a shallow cavity often causes tooth sensitivity. This frustrates both you and the doctor.

To treat sensitive teeth after a new filling is placed, a dentist often removes the new filling, places a sedative filling (usually, a zinc oxide and eugenol paste which hardens), and leaves the tooth alone for six to 10 weeks and then places a new perma-nent filling. Sometimes this helps, but sometimes it doesn't.

Today, many dentists won't place fillings which contain mercury (called *amalgams*). The newer composite (tooth col-ored, plastic-like fillings) are beautiful and mercury-free, but they often produce severe thermal sensitivity. In the process of placing composite fillings, dentists use a gel material (phos-phoric acid) to etch the edges of the enamel to improve the retention (or, holding) and sealing of the filling. If any of this acid accidentally touches the underlying dentin, the tooth's pulp is chemically damaged, producing cold sensitivity. This irritation usually subsides in a few weeks, but in some people, the sensitivity may last months or years. This is especially true if the cavity being fixed is deep.

What can you do for teeth sensitive to cold tempera-tures after dental treatment? Talk with your dentist. Sometimes adjusting the occlusion (bite) corrects the prob-lem. I often prescribe aspirin or ibuprofen for about 10 days and have the patient avoid any extremes in either hot or cold temperatures.

After the placement of a new filling or crown, you may notice you're clenching your teeth. Some people develop oc-clusal awareness, or an unnatural awareness of the teeth, and this generally causes one to clench or grind, producing sensi-tive teeth. Adjusting the tooth, new filling, or using a mouth guard at night usually reduces the sensitivity.

There are times when you'll never be rid of thermal sensitivity. I have this problem with a crown placed in 1977. I've had other teeth crowned since then which have no thermal sensitivity, so I

Have patience with your dentist if you develop this problem. It's frustrating him, too.

know as a patient what it's like to suffer tooth pain from cold temperatures. There are worse problems in life, but sensitive teeth are irritating. Have patience with your dentist if you develop this problem. It's frustrating him, too.

Malocclusion

You might develop malocclusion, or an improper biting of the teeth, after your dentist places a new filling, crown, or partial denture. When numb from the local anesthetic, you can't bite properly for a few hours. Your dentist uses articulating paper (a type of carbon paper that shows how you're biting) to check your occlusion. At first you'll think the occlusion feels funny because of the new restoration . . . and that may be the case. But if your occlusion isn't correct (you can detect as little as one-ten thousandths of an inch in you bite), you'll begin to grind, clench or simply bite improperly and you'll develop sore and sensitive teeth, headaches, earaches, and jaw and TMJ pain.

Go back to your dentist and have your occlusion evaluated. Usually, he'll slightly adjust your occlusion and you'll be fine. You may have to return a couple of times, especially if you received several fillings or crowns.

Your dentist may need to make an occlusal splint (a special mouth guard) to relax your muscles before he can adequately adjust your occlusion so that you're comfortable. This isn't often necessary. If your dentist wants to adjust several teeth, demand a splint to relax your muscles or else too much tooth structure may be removed.

Table 4.1: Common causes of odontalgia									
Causes of Pain	Tooth Decay	Tooth Abscess	Cracked Tooth	Exposed Root	Maloc-clusion	Broken Filling	New Filling	Wisdom Tooth	Perio-dontal*
Heat	Some-times	Yes	Some-times	Usually no	No	Some-times	No	No	No
Cold	Some-times	At times	Yes	Yes	Yes	Yes	At times	No	Often
Touch	No	Often	Yes	No	At times	No	No	No	No
Biting	At times	Yes	Yes	No	Yes	Often	At times	Some-times	Some-times
Lying Down	No	Yes	No	No	Often	No	No	Some-times	Some-times
Hard Foods	Some-times	Yes	Yes	No	Yes	Some-times	Some-times	Some-times	Some times
Sweet Foods	Yes	No	Yes	Yes	No	Some-times	No	No	No
*Periodontal pain: see Chapter 5.									

Impacted Teeth

First, what's an impacted tooth? We use that term all the time, but what does it really mean? Basically, an impacted tooth is one that's confined or trapped within the jaw bone or gingival (gum) tissues.

Impacted teeth occur most often in the third molar, or wisdom tooth, areas (Figure 4.6).

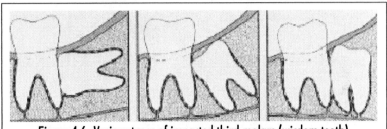

Figure 4.6: Various types of impacted third molars (wisdom teeth).

Yet, any tooth may be impacted. For example, maxillary (upper) cuspids are commonly impacted and we must surgically expose them so the orthodontist can attach a bracket to the tooth and move it into the proper position.

Impacted wisdom teeth may cause pain. Infections, cysts, obstruction of surrounding teeth, tumors, and periodontal defects occur around impacted teeth more often than around other teeth. That's one of the reasons your dentist takes a panoramic x-ray (the type that goes around your head) every few years. One of the structures he or she is watching are impacted teeth. For example, if a cyst develops, you rarely feel pain until much of the jaw bone is destroyed. That often causes dangerous problems, so just monitoring impactions is important.

Also, a partially impacted tooth often allows food to be trapped between it and a tooth in front of it. Cavities and periodontal problems develop and if not treated, teeth are destroyed and lost. Damage from an impacted tooth is one more reason to see your dentist on a regular basis.

Pain from impacted teeth is dull and diffuse, spreading beyond the area of the offending tooth. The pain, which occurs spontaneously, lasts for days or longer. It's not affected by temperatures or chemicals (e.g., sweets), but we do find pain when adjacent teeth are tapped.

Developing pain in nearby muscles is a big problem in diagnosis of this kind of pain. To make matter worse, if you have large fillings, fractured or worn teeth, the diffuse pain of an impacted tooth mimics muscle pain.

Impacted teeth also, at times, cause a pressure sensation in adjacent teeth and some orthodontists believe this pressure from impacted wisdom teeth causes all the teeth to move forward, thus crowding the front teeth, ruining all the wonderful orthodontic treatment. Statistically, we're not sure if this really happens, so listen to your dentist and orthodontist.

Have you ever known an adult who complained of a tooth erupting? Impacted teeth have the potential to erupt any time in life, no matter the patient's age.

Because pathological problems occur often in association with impacted teeth, we often recommend surgical removal of these time bombs, especially when the patient is young and healthy.

Teething Pain

What parent hasn't spent many sleepless nights, walking and rocking a baby suffering from the pain of teething? As parents, there's little we can do but suffer with the babies.

It's hard to believe, but some authorities actually doubt if babies experience pain when teething! Until recently, scientists have grossly neglected the idea that babies recognize pain. The major problem is the child's limited means of expressing pain. Doctors and nurses make an awful mistake when they confuse frozen terror and learned helplessness with quiet acceptance by babies. Obviously, these so-called experts have no children.

Why do erupting teeth cause pain? There are a couple of reasons. First, the act of an erupting tooth, slowing moving through bone and then breaking through the gum tissues obviously causes inflammation and subsequent pain.

Also, at times, an acute infection occurs when the gum tissues open-up as the tooth breaks through. Rarely does this cause a serious infection or problem, but still, in a little one who's only a few months old, even mild pain becomes a major problem . . . at 1:00 A.M. in the morning!

Parents associate high fevers, diarrhea, runny nose and skin rashes with teething. Most likely, these symptoms could signal more serious illnesses. Speaking as a doctor, none of these symptoms are connected with teething. As a father, however, I soon realized the textbook writers weren't always correct. However, common teething symptoms include:

- Drooling and excessive saliva
- Pain
- Mild, stuffy nose
- Bluish swollen areas in the gums
- Mild bleeding
- Occasional low-grade fever
- Fussiness like sleep or personality disturbances
- A fierce tendency to bite objects
  (watch out nursing mothers!)

What can you do to reduce the pain when your baby's teeth erupt? Chewing on a chilled, rubber-type toy or teething ring helps. Liquid acetaminophen as directed in the bottle's instructions really helps, but it takes time to work. Rub a little local anesthetic (e.g., Orajel) available from any pharmacy on the gum tissue directly over the erupting tooth. Gels work faster than liquid medicines. Even just rubbing your baby's gums with your clean finger is very comforting.

Some herbal remedies like clove oil, a natural anesthetic, work well. Talk to health food store employees or homeopathic practitioners about clove oil and other remedies.

Never put your child to bed with a bottle filled with milk, juice, or any liquid with sugar. You'd think this would be a comfort, especially when teething. But developing such a habit can lead to serious destruction and loss of all teeth before the child is 3 year old. This is tragic and avoidable.

Don't forget to clean your baby's new and existing teeth daily. As soon as teeth erupt, clean them daily with a wet wash cloth. Around age 10 to 12 months, brush the teeth daily with a wet tooth brush. Your child will not like this, but like most of parenting, consistency is the key. Don't use tooth paste until your child is around 2 years old. If you have any questions whatsoever, first, consult your family dentist.

Generally, in all generations since the Creation, parents have had to endure the inevitable event of tooth eruption. Like attitudes in teen-aged years, pain from tooth eruption will also pass.

Chapter Summary

Odontalgia has many causes. It's imperative that an accurate diagnosis be determined, or else irreversible dental procedures may be recommended. Far too many times I'm seen patients who've undergone numerous root canal procedures only to discover the actual diagnosis was malocclusion.

I can't emphasize enough that patients need to get additional opinions if their dentists aren't sure what's causing pain. Reputable and honest dentists will welcome the consultation advice of a colleague. Shouldn't the patient, and not the doctor's ego, be the focus of diagnosis and treatment?

References

1. **Wall PD and Jones M.** *Defeating Pain.* New York: Plenum Press, 1991.

2. **Murray PE, About I, Lumley PJ, Smith G, Franquin JC, Smith AJ:** *Postoperative pulpal and repair responses.* J Am Dent Assoc 2000;131:321-329.

CHAPTER Five

Periodontal Pain

The word periodontal (peri = around; dontal = teeth) refers to the surrounding tissues, or ginginva (gums) and bone, around the teeth. Periodontal disease, then, is a disease that attacks the periodontal tissues. This disease is a broad category of several, similar, diseases.

Diagnosed in well over 80 percent of adults world-wide, periodontal disease affects an estimated 50 million Americans. Known as pyorrhea years ago, this gingival disease is the leading cause of tooth loss in adults. But children aren't protected from periodontal disease. Studies indicate the prevalence of periodontal disease is 1% to 9% of 5 to 11 year olds and anywhere from 1% to 46% in 12 to 15 year olds.

Several clinically distinct infections, all collectively termed periodontal disease, affect all ages of human beings. The most notable are: gingivitis, early onset periodontitis, generalized periodontitis and acute necrotizing ulcerative gingivitis. We'll explore the evidence that periodontal disease may contribute to systemic diseases.

Microorganisms

Over 500 microorganisms are known to cause periodontal infections. These infections are predominantly anaerobic (an = lack of; aerobic = oxygen). Many scientists believe the anatomic closeness of these bacteria to the bloodstream produce bacteremia (bacteria in the blood) and systemic spread of bacterial by-products. Clinical procedures such as tooth extraction, periodontal and endodontic (root canal) treatment, enable these microorganisms to enter the blood from the oral cavity. The microorganisms that gain entrance to the blood circulate throughout the body, but are usually eliminated by the body within minutes.

However, in patients with ineffective heart valves or vascular diseases, bacteremia is a potential danger, leading most commonly to infective endocarditis (infection of parts of the heart) and myocardial or cerebral infarction (heart attack and stroke, respectively). Other forms of systemic diseases such as brain abscesses, blood and implant infections have also been related to oral microorganisms.

Gingivitis

The first stage of periodontal disease is termed gingivitis, or inflammation of the gingiva. Hundreds of types of bacteria in the saliva produce a sticky substance known as plaque. Within the plaque, bacteria, food debris, and white blood cells are trapped. The bacteria produce toxins, stimulating the immune system, causing inflammation of the gingival tissues, thus producing gingivitis.

Gingivitis is a progressive disease, meaning that in the early stages, few if any indications of disease appear. The first symptom of gingivitis is bleeding gums when you brush or floss.

Gingivitis is a progressive disease, meaning that in the early stages, few if any indications of disease appear. The first symptom of gingivitis is bleeding gums when you brush or floss. Because there's no pain involved with gingivitis, most people aren't aware they have a disease of the periodontal tissues.

As the disease progresses, a stronger immune response is launched by the body, producing swollen and red gums. At this point, pain is still absent or very minor, but the gums bleed quite a lot when brushed. Your toothbrush will stain red from the bleeding. Fortunately, you can easily stop the infection by simply improving your oral hygiene, seeing your dental hygienist, and taking vitamins C , E, Coenzyme Q10, and the zinc gluconate. But gingivitis is a potentially serious problem because it rapidly changes to chronic periodontal disease usually without any pain.

We easily treat gingivitis by using good oral hygiene techniques, routine dental cleanings, dietary changes, and taking nutritional supplements.

Early Onset Periodontitis

Early onset periodontitis is a rare, distinct type of periodontal disease that affects young individuals who are otherwise healthy. Also termed juvenile periodontitis, teenagers and young adults are affected. These patients often don't suffer first with gingivitis as do adults. This type of periodontal disease is self-limiting if confined to a single area (termed localized juvenile periodontitis). If most of the periodontal tissues throughout the mouth are involved (termed generalized juvenile periodontitis), there's a rapid rate of destruction of the bone and gum tissues around permanent teeth. As you can imagine, this is a severe and debilitating disease, often leading to partial or even complete tooth loss in teenagers and young adults.

Unlike older patients afflicted with periodontal disease, those with localized juvenile periodontitis rarely form dental plaque or calculus (tartar). Apparently, this form of periodontal disease is caused by very aggressive bacteria, defects in certain white blood cells, or both.

Generalized juvenile periodontitis usually starts around puberty. Unlike patients with the localized type, individuals with the generalized form have severe periodontal inflammation (with much bleeding) and heavy accumulations of plaque and calculus.

Early onset periodontitis is best treated with a combination of antibiotics (tetracycline works best) and periodontal surgery to correct the defects caused by the disease process. We also teach patients good oral hygiene techniques.

Periodontitis

As gingivitis proceeds, it develops into periodontitis, which means the gingival and bone tissues are infected. Pockets form around the teeth eroding the bony support of the teeth. A tooth is like a fence post: its root is buried deep within the jawbone like the post is buried deep in the ground (Figures 5.1 and 5.2). However, as water, wind, snow and ice wear away the dirt around the fence post, it ultimately becomes loose. Teeth loosen, too, as the bacteria, both aerobic (bacteria which must have oxygen to live) and anaerobic (bacteria which die in the presence of oxygen) and inflammation wear away the periodontal structures.

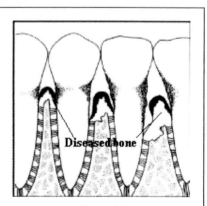

| Figure 5.1: | Figure 5.2: |
| Healthy periodontal tissues. | Diseased periodontal tissues. |

As bone is lost and teeth loosen, you'll feel pain throughout the gums and deep in the jawbones. Unlike pulpal or tooth pain, periodontal pain is more localized, easier to locate the source of pain. Your breath will smell horrible and, if you don't smoke or eat a lot of spicy foods, your mouth will also taste rancid.

The seven characteristic signs of periodontitis:

- Red, puffy gums

- Bleeding gums

- Persistent bad breath

- Spaces that develop between teeth

- One or more teeth become loose

- Receding gums (your teeth will look longer)

- Aching, itching or pain in the gums

Severe periodontal disease often makes the sufferer feel ill all over. When I was an army corpsman, we stressed good oral hygiene techniques more than any other type of personal hygiene because periodontal disease could quickly incapacitate soldiers in the field, especially in the jungle. Military doctors and commanders knew that an effective army couldn't afford to suffer from periodontal problems and remain alert and effective.

Is periodontal disease communicable? Yes, like colds, you can catch periodontal disease from someone who's infected. The American Dental Association estimates 20 to 30% of spouses pass periodontal disease to their spouse. There's even evidence of transmission of periodontal disease in caring for a child. But kissing isn't the only way to pass bacteria which cause periodontal disease. Using the same drinking glass or food utensils spread bacteria among people.

While there's no known cure for periodontal disease, it can be prevented by:

- Brushing and flossing properly to remove all plaque

- Seeing your dentist or dental hygienist for regular periodontal examinations and routine prophylaxis (dental cleaning)

- Eating a healthy diet

- Taking vitamins and mineral supplements

Each time you see your dentist or dental hygienist for a routine cleaning, the doctor or hygienist should examine all the tissues of your mouth and measure the depth of any pockets around your teeth. By checking the pocket depths and taking specific x-rays, periodontal disease is easily detected.

We treat periodontal disease with a combination of improved oral hygiene, root planning and curettage (surgically scraping the gingiva), oral rinses, and occlusal adjustment (adjusting the bite). Root planning and curettage is a surgical procedure we use to smooth the roots of the teeth and eliminate the pockets around the teeth. If these techniques don't halt periodontal destruction, more aggressive surgery is required.

Oral rinses are important in treating periodontal disease. Some doctors recommend Listerine mouthwash while others prescribe medications like Periodex. These chemicals kill certain bacteria which we believe are the prime causes of periodontal disease. I've also been impressed with the reduction of inflammation in oral rinses and tooth paste with tea tree oil. The results of aloe vera are also encouraging.

Many scientists believe that malocclusion, in the presence of periodontal disease, accelerates the destruction of the bone around the teeth.

Remember our discussion about trauma from occlusion in the last chapter? Many scientists believe that malocclusion, in the presence of periodontal disease, accelerates the destruction of the bone around the teeth. Therefore, most periodontists (a dentist who specializes in the diagnosis and treatment of periodontal diseases) adjust a patient's occlusion to lessen lateral forces on periodontally affected teeth.

I prescribe a mixture of baking soda, peroxide, a little salt, and a few drops of mouthwash to form a tooth paste. These ingredients all decrease gingival inflammation by killing various types of bacteria which multiply in the pockets around the teeth.

I also suggest taking the following supplements for any inflammatory problem, especially periodontal disease:

- Vitamin C: 2,000 mg to 4,000 mg per day
- Vitamin E: 400 IU twice daily
- Zinc gluconate: 50 mg to 100 mg daily
- Coenzyme Q10: 90 mg to 150 mg per day
- Calcium: 800 mg to 1200 mg per day
- Magnesium: 600 mg to 900 mg per day
- Grapefruit seed extract
- Vitamin B complex
- Aloe vera rinses
- Odor-free garlic

Acute Necrotizing Ulcerative Gingivitis

Although considered rare, I've seen acute necrotizing ulcerative gingivitis (ANUG) in my practice several times. This periodontal disease is characterized by progressive and rapid inflammatory destruction of the gingival tissues and then the underlying bone.

At first, the gingival tissues between the teeth (termed interdental papillae) enlarge and bleed profusely. These soft tissues next develop ulcers, a tacky membrane, and ultimately, the gingival tissues die (become necrotic), producing crater-like ulcers in-between the teeth. This disease has a trait which alerts nearly any dentist as to the diagnosis: a horrible, fetid smell. Imagine the smell of dead, rotting tissues within a dark, moist environment like the mouth. Once you smell ANUG, you'll never forget it.

ANUG has been described in the literature for centuries and has been know by many different names: stomatitis, Vincent's stomatitis and trench mouth. It's been associated with stress, smoking, but especially with poor oral hygiene followed by an infection of specific bacteria. ANUG was a detrimental factor of soldiers in World War I, as many of them had no chance to brush their teeth. Coupled with the horrible stresses of wartime, heavy smoking and lack of proper sleep and nutrition, many of these brave men (on both sides) developed ANUG. The term trench mouth was coined in WWI because many of the soldiers in the trenches developed this oral disease.

The symptoms of ANUG are:

- Painful gums
- Profuse gum bleeding with any pressure or irritation to the gums
- Red, swollen gums
- Fever
- Weight loss
- Sore throat
- General malaise (feeling horrible all over)
- Grayish film on the gums
- Horrible smell
- Foul taste
- Crater-like ulcers in-between the teeth

We treat ANUG by controlling the infection locally in the mouth. The dead tissues have to be removed with both surgical instruments and with an ultrasonic cleanser. Frequent salt water and hydrogen peroxide rinses (first salt water and then peroxide) several times a day are effective in quickly controlling the infection. Also, we prescribe antibiotics, pain medication, and instruct the patient in proper oral hygiene techniques.

We encourage patients with ANUG to stop smoking and seek counseling concerning their stress. Patients also benefit from proper diet, rest and exercise.

If left untreated, ANUG will spread to other areas of the mouth, lips and jawbones, finally destroying these structures. Although rare, ANUG is not an infection to be ignored.

Periodontitis Associated with Systemic Disease

Until recently, the dental profession and research scientists paid little attention to the impact of periodontal infections on the human body. This is probably due to advent of antibiotics. Doctors thought they controlled periodontal infections by simply prescribing antibiotics. But did they?

In the late 19th and early 20th centuries, the Focal Theory of Infection was popular. At the beginning of the 20th century, William Hunter, an English physician and pathologist, in his article, The Role of Sepsis and Antisepsis in Medicine named the gold crown, ". . . a mausoleum of gold over a mass of sepsis."

According to this theory, foci (localized areas) of infections were responsible for such conditions as inflammatory diseases, arthritis, peptic ulcers, heart problems, and many other systemic diseases. Bacteria were thought to be carried from these foci of infections, through the blood stream, to these distant areas of the body. After antibiotics were invented, the Focal Theory of Infection was abandoned because the effects of wandering bacteria could be covered up with antibiotics.

The theory of focal infection played a dominating role in medicine for approximately 25 years (1907-1937), leading to widespread extraction of endodontically compromised teeth, and a virtual disappearance of endodontic therapy in the United States. During the next decades, with improvement in endodontic therapy, a total unconcern for focal infection developed among dental professionals. However, recent progress in oral pathology and the possibility of tracing organisms in extra-oral (outside the

Recent progress in oral pathology and the possibility of tracing organisms in extra-oral (outside the mouth) sites back to the oral cavity, have led to renewed interest in and concern for bacteremia and its systemic risks.

mouth) sites back to the oral cavity, have led to renewed interest in and concern for bacteremia and its systemic risks. In fact, the increase in organ transplants and the placement of implants today have caused the medical community to revisit and reconsider this disease theory.

Eating, flossing, tooth brushing, and tooth picking release bacteria (called bacteremia) regularly into the blood stream. During oral surgical procedures, bacteremia rises to an alarming rate. Why do you think physicians demand that their patients with implants, transplants, and heart problems take antibiotics before any dental procedure? Because they, organized medicine, the American Heart Association, and implant surgeons all believe in the Focal Theory of Infection, even if they won't admit it. If this abandoned theory of infection didn't have some validity today, then why do potential transplant patients have to perform meticulous oral hygiene procedures and be certified by a dentist that their oral tissues are healthy?

My beliefs about the Focal Theory of Infection were confirmed one day when I took one of my 9 dogs to the veterinarian. A couple of diagrams on the walls of the examining room described the Focal Theory. When I asked the vet if he really believed that dental diseases could cause systemic diseases, he simply asked, "Don't you human doctors believe that?" That comment was enough for me.

The two common systemic diseases associated with periodontitis, even by traditional physicians, are diabetes mellitus and cardiovascular diseases. Unfortunately, there are many others.

Diabetes. Insulin dependant diabetes mellitus (IDDM), or type I diabetes, is also called juvenile diabetes because it often occurs in young people. However, it can occur at any age and comprises about 10% of all cases of diabetes. Classic symptoms are frequent thirst, frequent eating, and frequent urination. The pathological problem is a lack of production of insulin because the insulin-producing cells in the pancreas (called, beta cells of the Islets of Langerhorn) have been destroyed by disease.

A second major form of diabetes is non-insulin dependent diabetes mellitus (NIDDM). This type of diabetes has also been termed adult onset diabetes. Treatment often consists of dietary changes and the use of very little, if any, artificial insulin. The pathological condition with this type of diabetes is a resistance of target tissues to the action of insulin.

Traditional medicine and dentistry freely admit to the association between diabetes and periodontal disease. In the past, periodontists realized that patients with diabetes had a greater tendency to have periodontal disease. Current scientific evidence shows that periodontal disease may influence the severity of diabetes, or at least, it may be a risk factor in the progression of diabetes.

Diabetic patients know that with time, they have a likelihood of developing degenerative eye and blood vessel problems. We know the underlying mechanism of these injuries is elevated glucose (termed *glycosylated hemoglobin*). Periodontal disease increases the blood glucose concentration and recent scientific studies have revealed that elimination of the periodontal disease lowers blood glucose levels. Diabetic patients must see the dentist or dental hygienist faithfully, often 3 or 4 times a year.

Cardiovascular Diseases and Atherosclerosis. Atherosclerosis is a progressive degenerative condition involving large to medium-sized arteries. Cholesterol crystals, plasma proteins (for example, fibrin and fibrinogen), certain cells, and bacteria (some from the mouth) form globes of deposits (termed *plaque*), which either block blood vessels or are the source of blood clots. Atherosclerosis with resulting blood clot formation producing loss of oxygen to the heart (ischemic heart disease) and stroke are the leading cause of death in the United States.

Further, classical risk factors of cardiovascular disease (CVD) (high blood pressure, elevated blood cholesterol and cigarette smoking) only account for one-half to two-thirds of CVD cases. Does periodontal play a role in CVD?

Statistically, there's a direct association between periodontal disease and CVD and strokes. Whether it's the bacteria themselves or their toxic by-products doesn't matter. The point is this: Periodontal infections, as regarded before the advent of antibiotics, appear to influence and perhaps produce cardiovascular diseases and cerebral strokes.

Other Diseases Associated With Periodontal Disease. Cardiovascular diseases, strokes and diabetes aren't the only systemic diseases which apparently are associated with periodontal diseases. Other diseases include:

- Infective endocarditis (bacterial infection of heart valves)

- Myocardial infarction (heart attack)

- Prosthetic heart valve infection

- Respiratory diseases, especially bacterial pneumonia

- Chronic obstructive pulmonary disease

- Organ abscesses

- Adverse pregnancy problems

- Joint implant infections

- Joint septic arthritis

- Low birth weight babies

Many homeopathic and naturopathic practitioners believe diseased teeth and periodontal tissues cause any number of systemic diseases, many of which are unnamed in this chapter.

Chapter Summary _____

Most adults throughout the world suffer with some form of periodontal disease. For the last 4 decades or so, the medical and dental communities have abandoned the Focal Theory of Infection, a theory which was held in high regard for two centuries until antibiotics were developed. Recently, scientists have renewed interest in the possible effects of periodontal disease throughout the body.

As a clinician and scientist, I find it interesting to observe that, as our population ages, more degenerative diseases appear and in general, with no known cause or causes. Could periodontal diseases and diseases of the teeth contribute to these diseases more than we've realized?

See your dentist regularly and practice good oral hygiene to reduce your risks of developing periodontal disease, especially if you have any other degenerative diseases.

References

1. **Johnson BD, Engel D:** *Acute necrotizing ulcerative gingivitis. A review of diagnosis, etiology and treatment.* J Periodontol 1986;57:141-150.

2. **Waldman BJ, Mont MA, Hugerford DS:** *Total knee arthroplasty infections associated with dental procedures.* J Bone Joint Surg Br 1999;81:56-59.

3. **Kim B, Weiss LP:** *Dentally induced bacteremia and infection of total joint replacement arthorplasty.* Focus Ohio Dent 1993;67:10-11.

4. **Scuderi GR, Scott WN:** *Total knee arthorplasty: What have we learned?* Am J Knee Surg 1996;9:73-75.

5. **Morrison HI, Ellison LF, Taylor GW:** *Periodontal disease and risk of fatal coronary heart and cerebrovascular diseases.* J Cardiovasc Risk 1999;6:7- 11.

6. **Mattila KJ, Valle MS, Nieminen MS, Valtonen VV, Heitaniemi KL:** *Dental infections and coronary atherosclerosis.* Atherosclerosis 1993;103:205-211.

7. **Mattila KJ:** *Dental infections as a risk factor for acute myocardial infarction.* Eur Heart J 1993;14 Suppl K:51 53.

8. **Loesche WJ, Schork A, Terpenning MS, Chen YM, Dominguez BL, Grossman N:** *Assessing the relationship between dental disease and coronary heart disease in elderly U.S. veterans.* J Am Dent Assoc 1998;129:301-311.

9. *Periodontal disease as a potential risk factor for systemic diseases.* A position paper. J Periodontol 1998;69:841-850.

10. **Debelian GJ, Olsen I, Tronstad L:** *Systemic Diseases Caused by Oral Microorganisms.* Endod Dent Traumatol 1994 Apr;10(2):57-65.

11. **Newman HN:** *Focal infection.* J. Dent. Res. 1996 75(12):1912-1919.

CHAPTER *Six*

Burning Mouth Syndrome

Imagine the frustration of having constant mouth pain. Not pain from a decayed or abscessed tooth, which you can isolate and treat. No, a constant pain throughout your mouth and tongue which interferes with eating and drinking, becoming progressively worse over time, has no known cause, and worst of all, rarely responds to treatment. Such is the plight of those suffering with burning mouth syndrome (BMS).

Clinical Features

We poorly understand burning mouth syndrome (medically known as *stomatodynia*). Patients usually complain of a burning sensation, which is more annoying than painful. Generally, the tongue, inside of the lips, palate, and the tissues covering the inside of the cheeks (termed the *buccal mucosa*) are affected. Patients with BMS describe their symptoms as a burning feeling as if the mouth were burned, on fire, or scalded. Many patients complain of bumps or at least the feeling of tiny bumps in the painful areas. They also often complain of a metallic taste even when they have no dental restorations containing metals. Acidic foods (citric juices, tomatoes, salsa), carbonated drinks, mouthwashes, and certain toothpastes cause considerable oral pain and a feeling of bumps developing. However, with most BMS patients, the oral tissues appear normal.

BMS effects over 2.5 million American adults, 25% being men.

Most patients (75%) with BMS are post-menopausal

women, but I've also seen several men with this problem. BMS effects over 2.5 million American adults, 25% being men. The burning sensations usually begin in late morning and peak by evening. As you might imagine, falling asleep is quite difficult, but once asleep, BMS patients aren't awakened with pain.

Some patients don't suffer with generalized mouth pain, only tongue pain, or *glossodynia*. These patients mostly complain of pain at the tip of the tongue or along the side or both sides of the tongue, all places of greatest rubbing against teeth or dentures.

Some researchers report a connection between BMS and some psychological disorders. For example, many BMS patients are very tidy, orderly, and often obsessive and compulsive. Further, these sufferers are often well-educated, and frequently their symptoms began with a change in social status. Before this upsets BMS sufferers, the most recent research does not prove any connection between BMS and psychological problems. Personally, I've seen obsessive/compulsive patients with BMS, but I've also seen many who were hardly tidy, orderly, or cared not one bit about their social status or appearance.

Another common characteristic of BMS is dry mouth or *xerostomia* and *dysgeusia* (altered taste perception). These patients suffer both with mouth burning and dryness.

Lastly, I've seen a few BMS patients whose pain began after his or her family dentist placed a metal restoration, especially when other, different metals were already present in other teeth. Through the electrically charged saliva, dissimilar metals work like battery terminals and generate an electrical current. You've probably sensed this very unpleasant sensation if you ever bit on a piece of aluminum foil or a metal fork. Imagine that feeling most of the time!

Diagnosis of BMS

There are no specific tests to prove or disprove BMS. So, we have to evaluate the patient's signs and symptoms. In addition, we look for a lack of other diseases and disorders. Biopsies are worthless for BMS. However, your dentist or oral surgeon may request a biopsy because an abnormality in the oral tissues might also be discovered.

It's important we rule-out a common oral disease: candidiasis (also known as thrust or simply a yeast infection). Candidiasis (mistakenly called Candida) is caused by an overgrowth of the yeast *Candida albacans*, a microscopic mold which is abundant in human beings. Candidiasis causes mouth burning, but the sufferer also sufferers with itching, reddening of the tissues, and at times, vaginal yeast infection in women. A simple and painless swabbing of the oral tissues will easily prove the presence of yeast. A frequent side-effect of aggressive antibiotic treatment, yeast over-growth is the most common problem which causes burning mouth and glossodynia.

A serious systemic cause of burning mouth is diabetes mellitus. Actually, the oral tissues are fine, but diabetics may develop a disorder termed diabetes neuropathy, which, at times, involves the oral tissues and tongue. Patients with BMS, frequent urination and intense thirst need to see an internist or family physician for a thorough evaluation to test for diabetes.

Other causes of BMS are:

- Gastric reflux
- Glucose intolerance
- Sjogrens disease
- Vitamin B complex deficiency
- Viral infections
- Parotid gland infections
- Central nervous system disorders

- Improperly cured denture material
- Allergies of metals in dental restorations
- Severe anxiety and stress
- Hormonal changes

Medications may be another cause of BMS. Certain drugs, especially the tricyclic antidepressive medications (see Chapter 12), produce a sideeffect, xerostomia. This dry mouth condition may, in turn, produce BMS. Other medications which induce xerostomia are muscle relaxants, diuretics, antispasmodics, antihistamines, anticonvulsants, antiarrhythmic drugs, and antihypertensives.

I've talked with many BMS sufferers who have one common cause or precipitating factor: a simple and routine dental prophylaxis or cleaning. One lady from Williamsport, Pennsylvania, emailed the following account to me:

> I've had this horrible disease since 1994. Actually I'm on the Internet this evening because it is so very bad yesterday and today. Nothing helps - only for seconds that is. Apple Juice soothes, but as soon as you swallow, the BMS is back. Pepsi, with it carbonation helps me, again only for seconds. I have most of the same symptoms as anyone else, however mine seems to affect my whole body. When BMS is bad, I feel as though I have the flu. Extremely tired, feel feverish (although I'm not). Sore throat (because the burning is so bad). I am just ill all over. Hope this helps you in some small way help others in your book. Actually I'm doing a lot of studying on this.

> There are a tremendous amount of patients with BMS that went to the dentist just before the onset !!! Very strange to me. I'm one of those people. Just had an ordinary checkup. The next day I woke up with BMS. Had it severely for about 12 weeks. If it would not have let up, I probably would have killed myself!!!

> Judy S. *(used with permission)*

I've seen and heard this story too many times not to believe it. Unfortunately, many of my colleagues immediately discount these reports either because they (the doctors) don't understand BMS, or they think the patient will hire an attorney and file a malpractice suit.

Treatment of BMS

Since we often can't identify the source of BMS, we aim our treatment at the symptoms. I've had good success using the drug Clonazepam, a medication usually used to combat convulsions. A recent scientific study of BMS patients who received Clonazepam revealed 43% of patients reported partial or complete relief of all symptoms, and a grand total of 70% experienced reduced oral pain. An added bonus is a return to normal taste for many of the patients in this study.

Reassurance helps in treating BMS. Understandably, some patients are very nervous when no one discovers the source of their burning sensations. Assuring a patient that he or she doesn't have a brain tumor or cancer is, at times, one of the best medicines we can offer. I also prescribe vitamin B complex and Nortriptyline or melatonin at bedtime.

Also, when symptoms escalate, I prescribe an oral rinse of topical anesthetic and anesthetic lozenges. Recently we've used hot, spicy candies (with cayenne pepper containing capsaicin), which is specially made to my prescription. Theoretically, the capsaicin makes the body initially produce many pain-producing chemicals, intensifying the pain at first. However, the production of these chemicals is soon exhausted and pain perception is dramatically reduced. This type of therapy is used elsewhere in the body to treat chronic pain. These results seriously suggest BMS is a problem of the peripheral pain pathways, meaning an actual and not psychological problem.

It's most important for anyone suffering with undiagnosed oral burning to see a dentist or an oral surgeon. Allow no one to perform an invasive procedure (such as surgery) without being sure of the diagnosis. As mentioned earlier,

BMS doesn't require surgical treatment and rarely, if ever, do BMS patients need a biopsy.

Also, realize BMS frustrates doctors as well. Be patient with your doctor if he or she is working with you to find the problem of BMS.

Lastly, I may refer a sufferer of BMS to a clinical psychologist to help them cope with this horrible disorder. I've seen many normal, healthy patients develop psychological problems such as heart palpitations, fatigue, being overly concerned about their health, and depression. These folks (and their family members) need encouragement and should talk to trained counselors.

CHAPTER Seven

Neuralgia Inducing Cavitational Osteonecrosis (NICO)

As recently as 1979, a newly described pain syndrome was reported by two separate researchers, Ratner and Roberts. This disorder, initially known as *cavitations* or Ratner bone cavities, produces pain similar to trigeminal neuralgia, both the typical and atypical types. In fact, usually these patients are first diagnosed with trigeminal neuralgia.

In 1992, a paper written by oral pathologist Dr. Jerry Bouquot was instrumental in changing the name to NICO (Neuralgia-Inducing Cavitational Osteonecrosis). In other words, pain due to dead bone which simulates trigeminal neuralgia. For years, orthopedic surgeons have been plagued with the problem of bone death in the head of the femur (ball portion of the upper leg bone). It now appears that bone in the jaws, especially the mandible, also develops this problem.

The diagnosis of NICO is not without controversy. For some strange reason, the dental profession refuses to believe these bony lesions exist. Yet, in orthopedic medicine, such lesions are a constant problem for the patient and surgeon alike. Why the dental profession and chiefly the oral and maxillofacial surgeons deny the existence of areas of dead bone is a mystery.

> *The diagnosis of NICO is not without controversy. For some strange reason, the dental profession refuses to believe these bony lesions exist.*

Every doctor, whether a dentist, oral surgeon, podiatrist, physician or orthopedic surgeon, was taught about the ravages of the conditions termed osteomyelitis and ischemic osteone-crosis. NICO is simply a variation of these conditions.

A early as 1915, Dr. G.V. Black, the father of modern dentistry, described these lesions in his pathology textbook, calling the condition chronic osteitis. Dr. Black felt this bony inflammatory process had the unique ability to produce extensive bone destruction without producing redness or swelling of the overlying tissues, without causing an increase in the patient's body temperature, and often without pain. He use the word cavity to describe these lesions within the bone marrow cavities. He recommended surgical curettage as an effective treatment. Later, this condition was known as osteonecrosis of the bone, often a direct result of osteomyelitis, or bone inflammation.

Osteomyelitis of the jaws was a very serious and life-threatening disease until the advent of antibiotics around the time the Second World War. Since then, such bony infections have been treated somewhat successfully with antibiotics. Yet, many of those afflicted with inflammation and subsequent dead bony area continued to suffer even with the use of antibiotics given intravenously.

Dr. Jerry Bouquot, an internationally renown oral pathologist (Past President of the American Academy or Oral Pathology and former Chairman of the Department of Oral Pathology, West Virginia University College of Dentistry) has not only described the condition of NICO, but he's linked this generic disorder to a multitude of causative factors, most of which are common with the development of bony lesions in other bones such as the femur (thigh bone). Approximately 20% of all hip replacements in the United States are due to ischemic osteonecrosis, so why wouldn't this disease effect the jaws as well? After all, the mandible and maxilla, like the femur, are medullary bones, meaning they contain blood marrow and produce blood cells.

Ischemic osteonecrosis isn't a disease in the usual sense but it's the result of a wide variety of local and systemic disorders that eventually lead to ischemia (lack of oxygen) and infarction (blockage of a blood vessel) of the vessels in bone marrow. In the jaws, the resultant disorder is termed NICO (Table 7.1).

Today, diagnostic techniques for NICO have never been better. In addition, today there are more dental surgeons treating osteomyelitis of the jaws than since G.V. Black's time. But the controversy continues, and many state dental boards are actively prosecuting dentists who attempt to relieve the pain and suffering of NICO or cavitation lesions of the jaws.

Causes of NICO

The cause of NICO seems to be similar to the development of dead bone in the head the femur: blockages in the tiny blood vessels, perhaps by the formation of blood clots due to a malfunction of one or several of the many steps in the normal clotting reaction. Apparently, minute blood clots form, thus preventing blood flow past the clot, thereby robbing areas of bone of oxygen. This process is similar to a stroke, blocking a tiny blood vessel in the brain, or a heart attack, robbing the brain or heart tissues of vital oxygen, causing death around the blockage (termed an *infarction*). In the jaws we think this problem of infarction plus the effects of

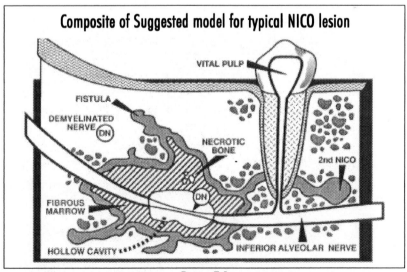

Figure 7.1

chronic bone inflammation from a dead tooth, an abscessed tooth, or poor healing after surgery are the causes of one or many areas of the bone dying, thus producing the symptoms of NICO (Figure 7.1).

Just to demonstrate that NICO isn't a figment of my imagination or that of Dr. Bouquot, Table 7.1 lists some of the suggested causes of jaw bone ischemia and infarction taken directly from the medical literature.

To date, we've isolated at least 73 causes or risk factors for the development of ischemic osteonecrosis. These factors ap-

Table 7.1: Factors suspected of causing ischemic osteonecrosis of the bone.	
Local Factors	**Systemic Factors**
Trauma (mild or severe)	Steroid therapy
Chronic tooth infection	Occupational atmospheric changes
Inadequate root canal treatment	Birth control pills
Bony infection/inflammation	Sickle cell diseases
Radiation therapy	Estrogen therapy—high doses
Swelling after oral surgery	Heavy smoking
Bone dysplasia	Thrombophilia
Constriction of blood vessels from local anesthetics	Antiphospholipid antibody syndrome
Implants which obstruct blood flow	Hypofibrinolysis
Injection of cortisone into bone	Systemic lupus erythematosus

ply to all bones, including the jaws. And we might ask, "Why not the jaws?" "Trauma and infection are the primary triggering events for this disease, and no other bones in the body come close to the amount of trauma and infection experienced by the jaws, from dental and periodontal infections, from tooth extractions, and from oral, endodontic and periodontic surgery."

Although we've isolated many probable causes of NICO, the most common I see are:

- **Trauma,** which may be mild or severe direct blows to the jaws;

- **Persistent tooth infections.** These may be as simple as a chronically sensitive tooth or a severe tooth infection which requires root canal therapy and even subsequent extraction of the tooth.

- **Surgical trauma.** Next to a history of chronic tooth pain, generally ending in removal of the tooth, I find bone trauma from simple removal of a tooth (especially 3rd molars), periodontal or endodontic surgery and other common dental procedures are quite common in NICO patients.

Symptoms

In some people, NICO lesions may produce no local symptoms, especially if we find no redness over the area or signs of drainage. However, in others, these lesions may produce intense, trigeminal neuralgia-like symptoms, which cause suffering to such an extent I wonder how some of these patients can stand it.

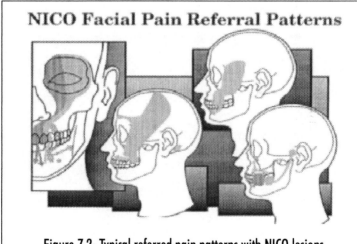

NICO Facial Pain Referral Patterns

Figure 7.2: Typical referred pain patterns with NICO lesions.

There are characteristic referred pain patterns (Figure 7.2), which I find consistent in most symptomatic cases. In those patients with pain, usually they have an underlying dull aching similar to atypical trigeminal neuralgia (Chapter 3). Along with this gnawing, deep pain, often there's a sharp, shooting pain which understandably convinces doctors that the diagnosis is trigeminal neuralgia.

Some patients have a fever and drainage into the mouth directly from the cavitation in the bone. This drainage produces a sour, persistent taste. This symptom makes many patients and doctors alike consider a diagnosis of sinusitis (Chapter 9), but unfortunately, all the sinus surgery in the world will not correct the problem if it's NICO.

To confuse matters more, many patients report systemic symptoms like arm or even leg pain or generalized fatigue. I'm seen several patients with symptoms of chronic fatigue syndrome which, once the NICO lesion or lesions were removed, dramatically improved.

There also seems to be a connection of yeast infection (termed *Candidiasis*) with many NICO patients. Why? I don't know, but when I've treated patients for yeast infections when they didn't respond well to surgery, many improved greatly. Perhaps the patient's immune system is compromised with NICO which leads to an over-growth of yeast throughout the body.

The typical NICO patient – and this is terrible – has his or her pain for approximately 6 years, before being properly diagnosed! Can you imagine the amount of money, suffering, lost work time, and family disruption these people have been through?

Are both the upper jaw (maxilla) and the lower jaw (mandible) affected with NICO? In a study conducted by Dr. Bouquot where he analyzed biopsy material from 2,301 NICO lesions, the maxilla was slightly more involved (51.5%) than the mandible (48.5%). However, in my practice, it's safe to say I see more mandibular lesions (perhaps, 70%) than maxillary ones.

Table 7.2 lists the proportion of sites of NICO lesions in Bouquot's study. You'll see the back of the jaw, where molars are located, seem to the most common areas of osteonecrosis. In my practice, the most common site is the mandibular third molar (wisdom tooth) region, followed by the mandibular first molar area and then the maxillary cuspid ("eye" tooth) region.

Needless to say, such a large study is convincing that there's a problem. And these results were all based upon microscopic examination of biopsy material. Regardless of what

Table 7.2: Distribution of NICO lesions based on 2,301 biopsies.			
Jaw Location	Maxilla (%)	Mandible (%)	Total (%)
Central incisor	2.5	0.2	2.7
Lateral incisor	3.6	0.2	3.8
Cuspid	5.0	2.0	7.0
First bicuspid	5.2	1.1	6.3
Second bicuspid	4.8	3.4	8.2
First molar	6.8	12.6	19.4
Second molar	2.6	5.1	7.7
Third molar	20.0	24.9	44.9
Total	51.5%	48.5%	100.0%

From: Bouquot JE, McMahon RE: Ischemic osteonecrosis in facial pain syndromes. Part I: a review of NICO. Morgantown: The Maxillofacial Center.

one may wish to think, NICO lesions are a real and devastating problem. As a friend of mine likes to say, "Your eyes only see what your brain tells them." Good wisdom!

Some of the more common symptoms of NICO are:

- Deep bone pain, which is constant but varies in intensity

- Sharp, shooting pain from the jaws which eludes doctors' diagnostic attempts

- Chronic maxillary sinus congestion and pain

- Pain which slowly progresses over time

- A sour or bitter taste, often causing gagging

- A history of a large filling being placed (or replaced), followed by pain, root canal therapy, and ultimately, removal of the tooth

- Failed attempts to treat trigeminal neuralgia

- A history of tooth removal years earlier

The most common scenario I see usually starts with a

tooth problem. Usually, a dentist replaces an old restoration and the tooth becomes sensitive, especially to cold temperatures. The filling may be replaced again, but the sensitivity persists. Then, in most cases, the tooth is treated with a root canal, but guess what? The pain continues. Another doctor is often consulted, only to have the root canal treatment repeated . . . and yes, the pain continues. Finally, out of sheer desperation, the tooth is extracted, only to have the pain continue and usually, intensify.

In the scenario above, the finest dentistry was performed, but something went wrong. It wasn't negligence by the dentist, but damage to the tiny vessels in the jaw bone around the injured tooth. Assaulted by constant inflammation and swelling, an infarction occurs in one or more of the tiny vessels, producing ischemic osteonecrosis. The result? A NICO lesion.

Diagnosis of NICO Lesions

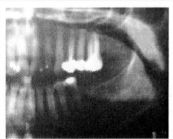

Figure 7.3:
Same panoramic x-ray as Figure 7.4 with NICO identified.

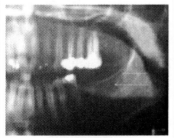

Figure 7.4:
Normal appearing panoramic x-ray.

The diagnosis of NICO is complicated by the fact that x-ray examination of the bone often appears normal. Considerable diagnostic experience is required because changes in the bone are subtle and may mimic a number of other entities, including variations of normal anatomy. Why is this so? Well, osteonecrosis is a disease of the marrow spaces and 30 to 50% of such bone must be destroyed before changes can be seen on x-rays. So if your dentist takes an x-ray and pronounces it normal in spite of your symptoms, he may be wrong. X-rays may mistakenly be interpreted as normal unless a significant amount of bone has been destroyed.

Like any other skill, the more you practice, the better you get. When I began treating NICO lesions in 1985 or so, I too, couldn't see cavitations on x-rays. Today, viewing the same x-rays, the cavitational lesions can't be missed.

Although MRI (magnetic resonance imaging) is the imaging of choice for osteonecrosis of long bones (e.g., the femur), flat bones of the face seem not to be imaged well with MRI scans. In fact, CT scans are also not successful in finding NICO lesions in the mandible or maxilla.

The best x-ray techniques for NICO lesions are (1) the panoramic x-ray (Figure 7.3) and (2) the periapical (routine dental) x-ray. The panoramic x-ray is the one your dentist takes to look at your wisdom teeth and sinuses. It shows all the jaws, maxillary and frontal sinuses, teeth, and portions of the temporomandibular joints. With experience, one can spot most NICO lesions from a panoramic x-ray (Figure 7.4).

In August 2001, the FDA approved the use of a new device, the Cavitat, which uses sonography to show NICO lesions in jawbones. Used in conjunction with a panoramic x-ray, we can now visualize the size and extent of these cavitations in two and three dimensions. You can believe how much the Cavitat has helped our diagnostic abilities and greatly improved our surgical success rates.

I can't imagine practicing without using this remarkable diagnostic tool. Panoramic x-rays are important, but a Cavitat scan is so helpful that I won't consider operating without a scan.

A useful way to diagnose painful NICO lesions is through anesthetic confirmation or anesthetic blocking. By giving a local anesthetic (similar to having your dentist numb the jaw before having a filling placed), areas in the jaws can be selectively turned-off,

> *The useful way to diagnose NICO lesions is through anesthetic confirmation or anesthetic blocking.*

meaning the sense of feeling (also pain) can be chemically and temporarily eliminated. If pain goes away after an injection, then both you and the doctor can be reasonably certain that there's a problem in the anesthetized area producing pain.

By adding this information to what we learn from a patient's history and by looking at the patient's x-rays, we can arrive at a fairly accurate diagnosis of NICO (if that happens to be the case).

A new ultrasonic instrument, the Cavitat, has been designed to send ultrasonic waves through the jaw bones. The information received from the ultrasonic scan is used to generate a 3-dimensional image of the bone outlining cavitational lesions. Currently, only a very few Cavitats are being used as they've only recently received FDA approval. In my experience, NICO lesions are most accurately diagnosed with the cavitat. I would not practice without this amazing device.

Electro-acupuncture through machines such as a Computron has been used fairly effectively for locating NICO lesions. Chiropractors and alternative medical therapists often use a Computron for many purposes. I work with a couple of chiropractors who are nearly 100% accurate concerning dead or dying teeth and the location of NICO lesions.

Treatment of NICO

A few different modes of therapy are used today in treating NICO lesions:

- **Antibiotics.** Prescribing antibiotics may temporarily reduce pain associated with a NICO lesion, but due to a compromised blood supply, not much of the antibiotic can actually get into and around the bony lesion.

- **Injection of homeopathic remedies.** Some doctors inject homeopathic remedies directly into NICO lesions. This will never work permanently. As much as I respect homeopathy, a doctor may inject anything into a cavitational lesion and observe similar results: nothing and often worsening of the condition. Remember, the bone within a NICO lesion is dead and has no blood supply to permit normal healing and removal of toxins and metabolites.

- **Anticoagulant therapy.** When a patient has a systemic clotting problem (e.g., fibrinolysis) along with other risk factors, we often use various anticlotting medications (e.g, Coumadin and low weight heparin) to prevent any further clotting within the bony blood vessels.

• **Hyperbaric therapy.** Through reports in the scientific literature, we think a combination of surgery, antibiotic therapy, and hyperbaric chamber therapy seems to have a slight positive effect on improving surgical outcomes.

• **Surgery.** *The only effective way to treat NICO lesions today is surgical curettage of the lesion itself,* removing the dead bone and marrow, and praying for new, healthy bone to develop in the defective area (Figure 7.5).

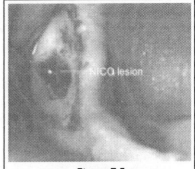

Figure 7.5:
Nico lesion in right posterior mandible as it appeared after incision and reflection (uncovering) of soft tissues.

A sample of material removed during surgery must be biopsied. The only true way to diagnose NICO or cavitational lesions is by evaluating this biopsy material through the microscope. Many bony disorders produce similar x-ray appearances to NICO, so a biopsy is needed to confirm or rule out the suspected diagnosis.

What about failures? I'm sorry to report that NICO has a strong tendency to recur and/or develop additional lesions about 33% of the time. Also, 10 to 12% have no or little pain reduction and about 15% have moderate improvement. Sadly, nearly 3% have an increase in pain after surgery.

Patients who don't respond to surgery often have multiple NICO lesions, a systemic yeast infection, or both. Recently, I've been treating all patients as if they had a systemic yeast infection, as everyone has when I've studied slides of their mouths under the microscope. Our success rate has climbed and patients have recovered quicker and better.

> *Patients who don't respond to surgery often have multiple NICO lesions, a systemic yeast infection, or both.*

If you're treated by someone for a NICO problem, be sure any material removed during surgery, including teeth (usually), be sent for biopsy to a pathology laboratory. This is very important in order to (1) establish the correct diagnosis and (2) to rule-out any other abnormalities which may be in the bone.

What Can You Do?

If you or a loved-one suspects a NICO problem, what can you do? First, allow no one, regardless of his or her number of degrees, to operate without first proving the pain can be stopped with a local anesthetic injection. If the pain can't be erased for a short time with a local anesthetic, chances are, there's another problem causing it.

Also, find a dentist who is both trained and experienced in the diagnosis and treatment of NICO lesions. There are few such doctors today worldwide. When finding a doctor, ask the receptionist the following questions when making your consultation appointment:

1. What type of training does the doctor have concerning NICO?

2. How long has the doctor been treating NICO patients?

3. What's his or her success rate? If you're told more than 70% or so, at the present time, find another doctor. We hope this will change soon, but today, 70to 75% success rate is standard percentage.

4. Who would the doctor suggest for a second opinion? If a doctor won't provide the name or names of other doctors for a patient to visit for a second opinion, then I'd suggest not making an appointment. If the diagnosis is correct in this office, it will be correct in another office, too.

5. How does the doctor use the cavitat? This is the best way, along with x-rays, to diagnose NICO.

6. Is the doctor a member of any medical academies? Although it's not mandatory, most NICO doctors are members of the American Academy of Craniofacial Pain, the International Academy of Oral Medicine and Toxicology, or both.

7. Does the doctor biopsy materials removed during surgery?

A Word of Caution

Due to the anatomical complexities of the mandible and maxilla, the possible post-operative consequences of NICO must be weighted against the benefits of surgery. Some of the possible post-operative complications include:

- Pain, bruising, infection
- Only partial improvment
- No improvement, or worsening of the pain
- Injury or invasion to the maxiallry sinus (upper jaw)
- Injury to the inferior alveolar nerve in the lower jaw, which may be permanent
- Tooth loss

True Story - *To all who suffer with facial pain!*

My name is Leslie Chill, a British expatriate who has lived in Southern California for the last 15 years. My story started 3 1/2 years (1996) ago after I had osseous surgery (a type of periodontal surgery). Approximately 2 to 3 weeks after the above event, I experienced extreme pain in my upper and lower left jaw.

This was the start of many visits to my dentist, periodontist, endodontist, regular doctor (MD), and neurologist. My diagnosis and treatment ranged from TMJ, root canals, to teeth extractions; none of which cured my pain and ultimately may have contributed to it. The neurologist diagnosed my condition as trigeminal neuralgia and initially prescribed Tegretol in low doses, but increased the dosage up to a maximum of 1600 mg daily. My pain did not subside. Then the dosage was combined with Neurontin at 300 mg daily as a last ditch effort to ease my pain. Finally, he recommended microvascular decompression (MVD) surgery (brain surgery).

It was at this stage (around September of 1999) that I could barely eat or speak due to the pain. I lost my job as a supervisor for a major auto parts company because I couldn't talk due to the pain. My German fiance Barbara, a former nurse, decided to investigate my condition through the library and Internet. Barbara eventually came upon Dr. Shankland's web site, where he described a little known disease called NICO, the symptoms of which described my condition exactly!!!!

We immediately contacted his office and after initial introductions, we emailed him a copy of a panorex x-ray that I had taken at his request. Dr. Shankland advised holding off on the MVD surgery and suggested I make an appointment to see him in Columbus, Ohio, as he saw signs of NICO on my x-ray.

We traveled to see Dr. Shankland in December of 1999. It was necessary for Barbara to talk for me because I was unable, and after the examination I had NICO surgery on my upper and lower left jaws. I had immediate relief following surgery and was able to talk without setting off the sharp pain. At that point in time I was taking a dosage of only 600mg Tegretol per day while my jaw was healing.

Since the surgery on December 13th, the pain in my upper jaw has all but disappeared. My lower jaw suffered a minor relapse at the end of December at which time we made another appointment to see Dr. Shankland on March 13, 2000. By the time we went to Columbus in March, my lower jaw had improved to the stage where I was only taking 200mg Tegretol combined with 600mg Neurontin per day. What a difference!

After an examination by Dr. Shankland, we decided to give the healing process more time, as it had only been 12 weeks since the surgery.

Needless to say, Barbara and I are both very grateful to Dr. Shankland for what he has done. It is so nice to be able to talk and eat once again without pain. Dr. Shankland has permission to give my home phone number to anyone suffering from NICO who would like to talk to me about my success story.

Chapter Summary

NICO lesions are real, regardless of what many dentists and oral surgeons may believe. These devastating areas of dead bone can produce intense pain which if often misdiagnosed as trigeminal neuralgia.

References (see Appendix B)

1. **Adams WR, Spolnik KJ, Bouquot JE:** *Maxillofacial osteoncrosis in a patient with multiple "idiopathic" facial pains.* J Oral Path Med 1999;28:423-432.

2. **Black GV.** *A Work on Special Dental Pathology.* Chicago: Medico- Dental Publishing Co, 1915:388-391.

3. **Bouquot JE, LaMarche MG:** *Ischemic osteonecrosis under fixed partial denture pontics: radiographic and microscopic features in 38 patients with chronic pain.* J Prosthet Dent 1999;81:148-158.

4. **Shankland WE:** *Osteocavitational lesions (Ratner bone cavities): frequently misdiagnosed as trigeminal neuralgia*–a case report. J Craniomand Pract 1993;11:232-234.

Eight

Craniofacial
Pain Disorders

Facial pain has many causes. When injured, many craniofacial (i.e., the head, face, and neck) structures refer pain to other areas, confusing both patient and doctor. Unfortunately, this confusion leads to inappropriate treatment, often worsening the patient's pain. That's why an accurate diagnosis is so important. If the doctor can't identify the problem, he or she takes a "shotgun" approach to treatment. Without determining the pain source, the doctor prescribes medication and therapy to no avail. In desperation and as a final resort, surgery is considered.

Many patients come to my office after multiple failed surgeries. A common thread intertwines all: the lack of a proper diagnosis.

Confusion concerning craniofacial pain disorders arises from a lack of medical training and an attitude that "it can't exist" if they (the doctors) didn't learn it in school. This is sad. We've discovered many pain disorders in the past 15 years that weren't (and still aren't!) taught in dental or medical school because the professors themselves weren't acquainted with them.

Before discussing pain disorders, let's distinguish between the terms disorder and disease. A disease is a pathological process, or abnormal condition, that displays classic symptoms. For example, if I mentioned "flu" or a "cold," you'd immediately know what I meant. Each of these viral infections have a specific set of symptoms (flu for example: fever, chills, muscle ache, nausea, etc.).

Disorders (syndromes), on the other hand, aren't so consistent. Not all symptoms must be evident in order to diagnose a disorder and not every sufferer exhibits all symptoms. This makes diagnosing of a disorder, as opposed to a disease, more difficult.

The disorders listed in this chapter have three important characteristics: (1) They produce pain and suffering to those afflicted; (2) they are frequently misdiagnosed, and therefore, usually improperly treated; and (3) they have little if any anatomical relevance to the temporomandibular joint (TMJ) other than a possible common embryological (developmental) origin. The last characteristic is important because many facial pain syndromes are mistakenly diagnosed as a TMJ problem and if the pain fails to resolve after routine treatment, joint surgery is often recommended.

Some of the more common syndromes or pain disorders are: Temporal tendinitis, Ernest syndrome, Eagle's syndrome, hamular process bursitis, sphenopalatine ganglion neuralgia, glossopharyngeal neuralgia, postherpetic neuralgia, Frey's neuralgia, and geniculate neuralgia.

Temporal Tendinitis

Generally, tendinitis simply means inflammation of a tendon. Tendons attach muscles to bones, with the tendons actually being embedded into the bone as a strong and resilient anchor for the muscle. Just imagine the forces on jaw muscles of a bear or lion when the creature bites into its prey. The jaw muscles must not only be strong, but the tendinous attachment into the bone has to withstand extreme pulling forces.

Temporal tendinitis is sometimes called "The Migraine Mimic" because many symptoms are similar to migraine headache pain.

We, too, have strong tendons, and the temporal tendon (also known as the temporalis tendon) is among the strongest and largest. The diagnosis of an inflamed temporal tendon is temporal tendinitis.

Temporal tendinitis is sometimes called "The Migraine Mimic" because many symptoms are similar to migraine headache pain. Dr. Edwin Ernest, my mentor and dear friend, first described this condition in 1983. The temporal tendon, a structure which attaches the temporalis muscle to the mandible at the coronoid process (Figure 8.1), produces approximately six specific referred pain patterns or painful areas when injured. Not all symptoms need to be present in order to establish the diagnosis of temporal tendinitis.

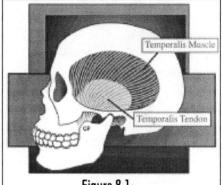

Figure 8.1:
Temporal tendon and temporalis muscle. CP = Coroniod Process

The temporalis muscle is one of the two major muscles that closes the jaw. The tendon is easily injured by trauma to the jaw, opening the mouth too wide, severe bruxism (grinding and/or clenching the teeth), or by building up the occlusion (bite) of the back teeth too high or too rapidly. Also, a displaced disc of the TMJ causes the temporalis muscle to contract abnormally, putting a great strain on the tendon. If this strain continues over a long period of time, a "tennis elbow" of the jaw occurs, producing severe TMJ-like pain. Chewing and wide opening of the mouth both worsen the symptoms of temporal tendinitis.

Table 8.1 lists the common referred pain areas from an injured temporal tendon. You'll learn in Chapter 14 the symptoms of a TMJ problem and then you'll see that the symptoms of temporal tendinitis are strikingly similar. That's one major reason why temporal tendinitis and TMJ are so often confused.

Misdiagnosis (or, more appropriately, missed-diagnosis) causes many unnecessary TMJ surgeries. Frequently the doctor treats a patient conservatively with the mistaken belief the diagnosis is a TMJ problem. If the pain refuses to respond to

TMJ treatment, the doctor refers the patient to an oral surgeon who, thinking conservative treatment a failure, performs TMJ surgery. Although the doctors try their best, the diagnosis and proper treatment of temporal tendinitis was never considered.

How do we diagnose temporal tendinitis? First, sufferers report many or all of the symptoms listed in Table 8.1. The symptoms that really alert me are stuffiness and/or a clogged feeling in the ear and temporal headache pain.

Second, we can confirm the diagnosis by injecting local anesthetic into the temporal tendon. If the pain and other symptoms subside after the injection, then both the patient and doctor can be reasonably sure the diagnosis is temporal tendinitis.

Table 8.1: Symptoms of temporal tendinitis.
TMJ Pain
Ear Pain & Pressure
Tooth Sensitivity
Cheek Pain
Eye Pain
Temporal Headache
Neck/Shoulder Pain

After the tendon is numb and if the pain complaints have subsided, we inject cortisone or Sarapin, a non-steroidal anti-inflammatory drug into the tendon. Then, we recommend physical therapy, which when used in conjunction with injections, it quite effective. Moist heat placed over the temple several times a day helps the healing process. If the patient bruxes at night, we make an anti-bruxism splint or an NTI appliance (Chapter 11).

If conservative treatment isn't successful, surgery is an option. However, as with TMJ surgery, consider these invasive approaches only as a last resort.

Temporal tendinitis often reoccurs, especially if a person is under a lot of stress and he's a bruxer or clencher. Understanding this, the patient may return for treatment once a year or so. However, at least he will have an idea what's causing his pain. Time and money won't be wasted looking for relief.

Zygomandibularis Tendinitis

A small but strong muscle, the zygomandibularis, attaches the skull to the mandible like the temporalis muscle through a long tendon. Chances are that none of your doctors have ever heard of this muscle because it wasn't reported in the scientific literature until 1995.

> *Chances are none of your doctors have never heard of this muscle because it wasn't reported in the scientific literature until 1995.*

Tendinitis of the zygomandibularis muscle occurs often with temporal tendinitis. In fact, many patients are successfully diagnosed with temporal tendinitis but when treatment is given and pain persists, the doctor and patient look elsewhere for another source of pain. They don't realize the zygomandibularis tendon is also inflamed, producing similar, but additional symptoms to the temporal tendon.

In addition to temporal pain, zygomandibularis tendinitis produces pain in and around the outside of the eye. Often, before I discovered this muscle while in graduate school, I'd inject the temporal tendon with a local anesthetic. The patient would receive maybe 80% relief of pain, but still, anterior temporal and eye pain persisted. Then, once I realized there were two tendinous structures producing similar symptoms, my diagnostic accuracy improved dramatically.

Like temporal tendinitis, patients with zygomandibularis tendinitis often have been hit in the jaw, had their mouth open for an extended period of time (for example, for a dental appointment or when being put to sleep for surgery), or are people who intensely clench their teeth.

Pain is felt deep to the corner of the eye. The pattern of pain almost circles the outside of the eye, and many sufferers think they have a sinus or eye problem. X-rays give us no help in diagnosing this tendinitis. The best diagnostic test is an injection of a local anesthetic directly into the tendon. This is very effective and, if the tendon is inflamed, stops the pain almost immediately.

Treatment for zygomandibularis tendinitis is similar to that of temporal tendinitis: injections of local anesthetic with Sarapin, a soft diet, physical therapy, and on NTI appliance (Chapter 11) to stop or reduce clenching.

In my practice, seeing the worst of the worst patients, I probably need to treat zygomandibularis tendinitis with radio frequency surgery 15% to 20% of the time. This in-office surgical procedure is very effective and safe. However, like most cases of tendinitis, re-injury to the zygomandibularis tendon is common and therefore, you may have to return to the doctor periodically for treatment.

Ernest Syndrome

In the early 1980s, Dr. Edwin Ernest first described a pain disorder that now bears his name: Ernest syndrome. This TMJ-like problem involves the stylomandibular ligament, a tiny structure that connects the base of the skull with the mandible, or lower jaw (Figure 8.2). When injured, this structure produces pain in as many as seven specific areas of the face, head and neck (Table 8.2).

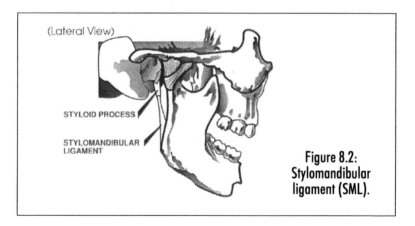

(Lateral View)

STYLOID PROCESS

STYLOMANDIBULAR LIGAMENT

Figure 8.2:
Stylomandibular ligament (SML).

The stylomandibular ligament prevents the lower jaw from moving too far forward. It also restricts the mouth from opening too wide by tightening when the lower jaw moves forward. Symptoms of an injured stylomandibular ligament are listed in Table 8.2.

Just like temporal tendinitis, Ernest syndrome's symptoms are frequently confused with symptoms of an injured TMJ. Sufferers will seek opinions from the family physician, ENT physician, chiropractors, but rarely do they consult a dentist.

The most common cause of Ernest syndrome is trauma to the lower jaw. Like whiplash injuries, direct trauma to the jaw isn't necessary. This painful condition may not be noticed for weeks or months after the injury, a common characteristic of soft tissue injuries.

Table 8.2: Symptoms of Ernest syndrome.
Temple Pain
TMJ Pain
Ear Pain
Cheek Pain
Eye Pain
Lower Molar Sensitivity
Throat Pain

The best test to see if the stylomandibular ligament is causing pain is to inject a small amount of anesthetic at the attachment of the this structure to the lower jaw. If the pain subsides after the anesthetic injection, the ligament is probably the source, confirming the diagnosis of Ernest syndrome.

Treatment for Ernest syndrome consists of repeated anesthetic injections followed with Sarapin injections into the ligament's attachment to the man-

Just like temporal tendinitis, Ernest syndrome's symptoms are frequently confused with symptoms of an injured TMJ.

dible. I also prescribe anti-inflammatory medications, moist heat, rest and a soft diet. This conservative therapy reduces or eliminates the symptoms of Ernest syndrome about 80% of the time. In those who don't respond to conservative therapy, we recommend surgery.

Initially, we treated Ernest syndrome by resecting (cutting) the stylomandibular ligament. We still use this procedure periodically, but it's dangerous because we can easily injure the facial nerve, which could produce paralysis of the facial muscles.

The most common and effective method we use to treat Ernest syndrome surgically is radiofrequency thermoneurolysis at the attachment of the ligament to the mandible. This is the same procedure described in Chapter 3 used to treat atypical trigeminal neuralgia.

A personal note. I was fortunate both to have been trained by Dr. Ernest and to be the researcher who conducted and published the first scientific study concerning Ernest syndrome. Prior to that time (1986), too many patients received inappropriate treatment and were misdiagnosed with Eagle's syndrome (see below), internal derangements of the TMJ, wisdom tooth problems, and trigeminal neuralgia.

Did these unfortunate persons suffer at the hands of negligent doctors who were only interested in making money? Not at all. But the diagnosis of Ernest syndrome is so new that only in the last couple of years have both the medical and dental communities accepted it. Still, many insurance companies won't recognize this disorder (Can you imagine that!). I have no doubt Providence arranged my friendship with the good doctor.

One patient from West Virginia had seen 19 doctors before seeing me. She complained of pain in all the areas listed above, and had received treatment for ear infections, cervical sprain, and TMJ problems. Fortunately, no one had yet operated. Listening to her complaints, performing a physical examination, and giving her a tiny anesthetic injection confirmed the diagnosis of Ernest syndrome. She ultimately required surgery.

Eagle's Syndrome

In contrast to Ernest syndrome, the malady most often associated with pharyngeal (throat) pain is Eagle's syndrome. Dr. Watt Eagle fully described this disorder in the 1930s. Unfortunately, most doctors, regardless of their degrees or specialties, confuse this syndrome with Ernest syndrome.

Dr. Eagle contended an elongated styloid process (Figure 8.3) or calcified stylohyoid ligament might cause severe pain and other throat symptoms. Eagle's patients fell into two categories: (1) those who had the symptoms of a foreign body lodged in the throat or (2) those who had neck pain along the distribution of the carotid artery, usually the external branch.

The styloid process (Greek: stylos, pillar or post; -oid: resemblance; therefore, a styloid is a bone resembling a pillar), is a small bone which descends off the base of the temporal bone on the base of the skull. The

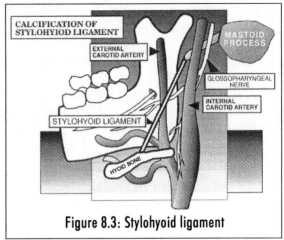

Figure 8.3: Stylohyoid ligament

stylohyoid ligament originates from the tip of the styloid process and ends by attaching to an area on the hyoid bone, a small bone in the front part of the throat. The stylohyoid ligament travels between the internal and external carotid arteries and just behind the back of the throat in the area of the tonsils.

The symptoms of Eagle's syndrome include:

• **A constant dull throat ache** which may be sharp and stabbing, **especially when swallowing** or turning the head

• **Ear pain,** which is usually deep and may even feel like an itch. The pain is dull but may be sharp at times, (which may also signal a TMJ problem).

• **Difficulty with swallowing.** Often, if the styloid process is elongated or the ligament which runs to the hyoid bone is calcified, swallowing may be irritating or even painful. Many times patients complain of feeling a chicken or fish bone caught in their throat. They clear their throats frequently and yet, the feeling of a foreign object remains.

• **Headache.** Eagle's syndrome often produces a dull temporal headache which intensifies when chewing.

The diagnosis of Eagle's syndrome is based upon the presence of the symptoms listed above, painful palpation (applying finger pressure) of a tender styloid process, and an elongated styloid process visible on an x-ray.

Radiologic (x-ray) viewing of an elongated styloid process is very important. The normal styloid process is visible with a panoramic x-ray, the one your dentist takes to examine your jaw bones and wisdom teeth. However, just because the styloid process is elongated doesn't mean that the diagnosis is Eagle's syndrome. A study of 1771 panoramic x-rays reported approximately 18.2% of the radiographs showed varying degrees of elongation of the styloid processes. No statistical correlations among increasing mineralization, age, and symptoms could be made.

To diagnosis Eagle's syndrome properly, I recommend that an anesthetic be injected into the area of the tonsils near the styloid process tip. This injection, given either inside or outside of the mouth, is complicated due to the vital deep structures of the neck in the vicinity of the styloid process tip (the carotid artery, for example). The injection is essential to differentiate Eagle's syndrome from Ernest syndrome, myofascial pain dysfunction of the posterior belly of the digastric muscle, or hyoid bone syndrome (see my first book: *TMJ: Its Many Faces*, 2nd edition. Columbus: Anadem Publishing, Columbus, 1998).

The only way to treat Eagle's syndrome is surgical resection (amputation) of the styloid process and/or the ossified stylohyoid ligament. Surgery is usually simple and can be performed either in the throat or from the outside, depending upon the surgeon's training. Usually, ENT doctors operate from the outside and oral surgeons from the inside of the throat.

Although rare, bilateral Eagle's syndrome does occur. Eagle's may also occur in conjunction with Ernest syndrome, especially after a severe traumatic injury.

Hamular Process Bursitis

The source of throat pain is one of the most difficult problems to diagnose and has been discussed in the medical literature for over a century, and until recently, we thought most throat pain was generally caused by the styloid syndromes, Ernest and Eagle's syndromes. But with several patients, I couldn't eliminate throat pain no matter how many times I injected the stylohyoid or stylomandibular ligaments. I knew there had to be another cause.

When I returned to graduate school to study anatomy, I purposely looked for any anatomical structure which might, when injured, contribute to throat pain. I found an answer.

Authors of anatomical articles mentioned the possibility of a tiny structure termed a *bursa*, on either side of the throat. A bura (Latin for sack) is a specialized tissue that produces synovial fluid, primarily in joints, to lubricate and nourish the surfaces of joints. Bursae also exist to reduce friction as tendons move around or over bones.

In the throat, two small bones extend down from the sphenoid bone on the base of the skull. These bones, one on either side of the throat, are the hamular processes. A strong soft palatal muscle, the tensor veli palatini, curves around these bones and tightly tenses the soft palate. For this mechanical activity, a bursa would theoretically be required to reduce the friction between the bone and the muscle. I was fortunate to be the first anatomist to prove the existence of this bursa.

Armed with this anatomical knowledge, I injected local anesthetic into these structures when I could find no other source of throat pain. And guess what? In many patients suffering with throat pain, the problem seemed to be an inflamed bursa of the hamular process.

The symptoms of bursitis of the hamular process are listed on the following page in Table 8.4.

Almost every sufferer of this bursitis reports consulting many doctors who could not end their pain. Frequently, pa-

Table 8.4: Symptoms of Hamular Process Bursitis
Soft Palate Pain
Throat Pain
Upper Jaw Pain
Difficulty Swallowing
Ear Pain
Redness Over Hamular Region

tients are wearing an upper denture, but only when in public, if worn at all, because the back end of the denture lies over the hamular processes. If inflamed, the pressure of the denture makes the pain worse.

We don't know the precise cause or causes of the bursitis. Trauma from swallowing a large mass of food or a denture which is too long seem to be reasonable causes. Also, some individuals simply have more prominent hamuli, making them more susceptible to mechanical trauma.

We diagnose bursitis of the hamular process by reviewing the symptoms and conducting a physical examination. But the real confirmation occurs if an anaesthetic injection into the hamular region stops the pain.

X-rays aren't helpful unless the hamular process is fractured. Inflammation of the bursa may be seen on an MRI, but this is difficult to see properly because of the small size of the hamular process and its associated bursa.

We treat bursitis of the hamular process two different ways. Most cases resolve simply by removing the trauma or irritation (e.g., adjusting the denture) and injecting synthetic cortisone into the hamulus region. I also prescribe anti-inflammatory medications.

If conservative treatment is unsuccessful, then we consider surgery. Performed under local anesthetic, the surgical procedure consists of amputating the hamular process. We've had good success with both conservative and surgical treatments.

Bursitis of the hamular process is such a newly reported disorder that most doctors, regardless of their degrees, know nothing about it. We can only hope that, in time, knowledge of this pain disorder will become more common.

Sadly, I've seen a correlation between hamular process bursitis and sexual abuse of an individual as a child. In cases like this, we need psychological and/or spiritual counseling as well as medical intervention.

Personal notes. David felt throat pain suddenly a few weeks after a sales trip to Houston. He couldn't recall any reason why his throat and ear bothered him until I asked if he'd been brushing his teeth vigorously and perhaps, slipped and hit his throat. "That's it!" he exclaimed. He was running late in the morning and while brushing his upper left back teeth quickly, his brush slipped and gouged his soft palate. Of course, it hurt him, but he had to arrive on time, so he thought nothing more about it. After returning home that night and having dinner with his wife, he noticed that his throat was sore on the left side. The pain persisted, so he saw his family doctor, who could finding nothing wrong but prescribed anti-biotics. His pain continued until his dentist referred him to our office. After injecting the hamular process area with local anesthetic, his throat and ear pain ceased. Ultimately, we had to operate and remove his hamular process, but today he's pain-free.

Another interesting case concerned a clinical psychologist who worked in pain management. The doctor, hailing from an East Coast state, was referred to my office with a history of a sore throat ever since he had undergone a general anesthetic for a minor surgical procedure. When he swallowed his pain intensified and worst of all, he was experiencing constant tinnitus (ringing in the ear) on the same side as his pain. I examined the doctor, and he quickly let me know that the hamular process was tender. I injected the bursa with local anesthetic, and within five minutes he was smiling, pain-free and, most astonishing to me, the tinnitus stopped as well.

When Mr. Smith came to my office, he carried a bag of dentures. He complained that his upper denture caused throat and ear pain and he only wore the denture to church and to shop. I soon discovered that he'd been in pain for over 40 years! He started having pain and kept seeing physicians and dentists, until one by one, all his upper teeth were removed, but to no avail. In addition, he had more dentures than an entire dental class could make in one year!

Here's the symptom that tipped me off: "I have no pain until I put my upper denture in. Then, my throat and ear hurt so bad that I can't wait to remove it."

I examined him and found both hamular processes tender. I injected both bursae with local anesthetic and left the room. When I returned in a few minutes, Mr. Smith was weeping. I couldn't imagine what I'd done. I began to apologize, and he immediately said, "No. No. This is the first time in over 40 years that I can wear my denture with no pain!"

I treated Mr. Smith with medications, and he responded wonderfully, and today, more than 15 year later, he's still pain-free.

Bursitis of the hamular process is such a newly diagnosed disorder most doctors won't know anything about it. We can only hope that, in time, the knowledge of this pain disorder will spread.

Sphenopalatine Ganglion Neuralgia

An unusual type of neuralgia is attributed to the spheno-palatine ganglion, which lies just below the maxillary division (or, second division) of the trigeminal nerve in an area termed the *ptygopalatine fossa*. This cave-like region is located deep within the skull, below and behind the nose. There are two such ganglia: right and left.

A ganglion is a collection of nerve cells, just like the Gasserian ganglion of the trigeminal nerve. In fact, the sphenopalatine ganglion is one of the four ganglia outside the cranium associated with the trigeminal nerve. Think of it as a relay station for sensory and autonomic nerves, which either begin in the ganglion or course through it on their paths to distant structures.

From the ganglion, nerves travel to the nose, eyes, sphe-noidal and ethmoidal sinuses, the hard and soft palates, the tonsils, throat, and ginginval tissues (gums) of the roof of the mouth.

Pain of sphenopalatine ganglion neuralgia (SPGN) is most likely due to a constriction of the blood vessels around the ganglion. Another cause may be a problem with the autonomic nerve supply to the ganglion. Whatever the cause, it's extremely painful and debilitating.

Sphenopalatine ganglion neuralgia is also known as Sluder's neuralgia, lower half (head) headache, and lower facial (midface and lower jaw) neuralgia. The pain is always on one side of the head. Symptoms of SPGN are listed in Table 8.5.

Table 8.5: Sphenopalatine ganglion neuralgia symptoms.
Nose pain, spreading to the eye
Pain in upper teeth, throat, ear, hard and soft palates, cheek
Temporal headache
Runny nose; tearing
Sneezing
Increased salivation
Sensitivity to light

The pain from this obscure neuralgia is so severe, patients literally bang their heads against the wall, hold their head, scream, and even beg to die.

Painful episodes can last from several minutes to hours. The pain is intense and described as burning and deep aching. Many sufferers' pain begin shortly after dental treatment on the upper teeth or after a maxillary sinus infection.

Diagnosis of SPGN is confirmed by numbing the sphe-nopalatine ganglion. We do this either by spraying a topical anesthetic through the nose directly onto the ganglion, or by injecting the ganglion with a local anesthetic through the roof of the mouth (the procedure I prefer). We have to make sure no any abscessed teeth or sinus infections, brain tumors, or temporal tendinitis exist. When severe, temporal tendinitis produces similar symptoms and may be misdiagnosed as SPGN.

We treat SPGN with medications and topical anesthetics. If the pain persists, then we consider surgical removal of the ganglion.

Some patients with SPGN who have a deviated nasal septum respond well after the deviated septum is repaired.

A personal note. When my receptionist saw my first SPGN patient, whose wife had driven him to my office, she immediately ushered him into a treatment room. His pain was so intense that he was nearly incoherent.

I immediately gave him an anesthetic injection to numb the spheopalatine ganglion which fortunately relieved his pain in a matter of a minute or so, thus confirming my diagnosis. It was like flipping an on switch off of a pain machine.

I attempted to treat him with medications and topical anesthetics. His condition improved, but still, his pain attacks continued. That's when I received the shock of my young professional life.

In an attempt to stop his pain, the man began using cocaine. That's right. By snorting cocaine, he unknowingly numbed his sphenopalatine ganglion and controlled his pain. When he confessed this illegal act to me, his guilt feelings were incredible, but what was he to do?

I'm happy to report that after consultation with a neurosurgeon, his condition was treated successfully and he abruptly stopped using cocaine.

Glossopharyngeal Neuralgia

This rare and distressing form of neuralgia is similar to trigeminal neuralgia. Many doctors regard it as a similar condition, but involving the glossopharyngeal nerve (the ninth cranial nerve) and the vagus nerve (the tenth cranial nerve).

It's hard to discover the cause of glossopharyngeal neuralgia, but generally it's due to pressure on the nerve by a blood vessel. At times, Eagle's and Ernest syndromes are misdiagnosed as ninth nerve neuralgia because of the severe throat pain all three conditions produce.

> *The pain of glossopharyngeal neuralgia is sharp, lightening-like, and lasts from seconds to a couple of minutes.*

Like typical trigeminal neuralgia, glossopharyngeal neuralgia's pain has triggers. The trigger areas are located in the tonsils, the ears, and on the base of the tongue. Primarily, any tongue movement (talking, chewing, swallowing, yawning, coughing or sneezing) or turning the head triggers the pain. The simple act of eating is torturous. Those afflicted with this syndrome lose weight.

The pain of glossopharyngeal neuralgia is sharp, lightening-like, and lasts from seconds to a couple of minutes. Remissions of the pain episodes occur, but tend to be shorter in duration. This is a terrible condition. The patients I've seen with this beg for any treatment, no matter how radical, just to receive some relief.

Since glossopharyngeal neuralgia's symptoms may mimic Eagle's and Ernest syndromes, it's important to determine the exact diagnosis. We first treat glossopharyngeal neuralgia with medications (like trigeminal neuralgia), and if that's unsuccessful, we consider surgery at the base of the skull.

Postherpetic Neuralgia

Most of us know the term *shingles*. The correct medical term, *herpes zoster*, is a painful disease caused by the herpes zoster (varicella-zoster) virus, which also causes chicken pox. Most cases of shingles heal completely and remain pain-free. Unfortunately, in about 20% of cases of shingles, pain continue as postherpetic neuralgia.

The common parts of the body affected are the upper torso, arms, or face. For most attacks, the acute phase lasts about a month. However, in older or sick patients, whose immune systems may be run-down, postherpetic neuralgia frequently develops into a chronic condition.

Rarely does postherpetic neuralgia occur before the age of 50. The incidence increases at a striking rate after age 60: At least 50% of people older than 60 years and nearly 75% of those beyond age 70 are affected after an attack of shingles.

We're not sure why, but it seems the herpes zoster virus lies dormant within the nerve ganglion until something activates it. Then shingles develops. Trauma and a depressed immune system are the two common factors which activate the latent virus.

Shingles first appears as a localized discomfort or tingling, with a skin rash developing within two weeks. The rash develops lesions throughout the distribution of the infected nerve. Pain sensations range from burning or itching to a stabbing feeling, and in a couple of days, fluid-filled skin lesions develop. The fluid is highly contagious and must be avoided by others. In some cases, the side of the face feels numb and weak, making chewing and talking difficult. Patients with shingles generally are fatigued and have a fever. These lesions seem to heal, but if pain continues, the condition is known as postherpetic neuralgia.

In the head, postherpetic neuralgia effects the ophthalmic division of the trigeminal nerve in two-thirds of cases. When the disease develops, the forehead and scalp remain sensitive after the skin lesions are gone. Washing, brushing or combing the hair, or a gentle touch of these areas causes intense, neuralgia-like pain.

Postherpetic neuralgia is difficult to treat. We generally prescribe Amitriptyline or Nortriptyline as soon as possible. I've also had reasonable success with prescribing cortisone, but this often treats the symptoms while the disease itself remains.

We also prescribe the medication Acyclovir, which helps the symptoms and seems to shorten the duration of the attack. Some alternative medicine doctors recommend taking L-lysine supplements, eating a high protein diet, and applying Zostrix (Capsaicin cream) topically.

A personal note. Forrest, who has become one of my favorite patients, has exacerbations of postherpetic neuralgia twice a year: when deer hunting and searching for mushrooms. Apparently, the cool air blowing over his face activates the sleeping virus, causing his forehead to break out with a bright red rash followed in a few days by large, fluid-filled lesions. His outbreak of shingles usually develops into postherpetic neuralgia, and that's when he sees me.

After talking about our hunting successes (or, lack thereof), I inject Forrest with a local anesthetic to stop his pain temporarily. Several times I've used radio frequency thermoneurolysis to deaden nerves, for as long as a year, that continued to cause pain.

Forrest still hunts deer and mushrooms, but at least he now covers his face, and this alone, has reduced the number of attacks of shingles. Consider doing the same if you develop shingles when you're enjoying nature.

By the way, I'm satisfied to receive from Forrest large, succulent mushrooms for payment of my services! Bartering isn't all that bad.

Frey's Neuralgia

This facial pain syndrome is foreign to most readers. It's rare, but we still see it, especially after TMJ surgery.

Frey's neuralgia (auriculotemporal nerve neuralgia) arises from damage to the auriculotemporal nerve. This large branch of the third division of the trigeminal nerve gives feeling to the TMJ, portions of the ear and parotid gland, and the skin of the temple. When we surgically enter the TMJ, we always injure the auriculotemporal nerve. Most of the time, only numbness over the joint and side of the head is the consequence of injury to the nerve. This usually lasts only 6 months or so.

Frey's neuralgia is an obscure pain syndrome which frequently is misdiagnosed as atypical facial pain. This neuralgia is characterized by unilateral burning, shooting pains in the side of the face, the TMJ, and the temple. When eating, the skin over the parotid gland turns red and the same skin perspires. Between episodes of chewing, the skin is very sensitive to touch.

The common cause of Frey's neuralgia seems to be trauma to the parotid gland either during child delivery (with forceps), blunt trauma to the face (e.g., hitting the side of the face on a steering wheel), or injury to the nerve supply of the parotid gland during surgery.

Treatment of Frey's neuralgia is challenging. The topical application of atropine-like drugs is sometimes effective. Cutting the auriculotemporal nerve often causes other problems like neuroma formation, an abnormal and painful growth of the stumps of cut nerves. This is usually more bothersome than the original Frey's neuralgia.

Some ENT doctors are using Botox (botulinum toxin) injections into the skin over the parotid gland. The long lasting results are impressive and safe.

Geniculate Neuralgia

Geniculate neuralgia is analogous to trigeminal neuralgia, except the seventh cranial nerve (or, facial nerve) is affected. The facial nerve provides movement to the muscles of the face, but a small portion of this cranial nerve also gives feeling to the ear, hard palate, and deep structures of the face. The division of the facial nerve that provides feeling is the nevus intermedius, so, this painful disorder is also known as intermediate neuralgia.

Symptoms of geniculate neuralgia include deep ear pain with a trigger area near the eardrum and pain radiation into the throat, face, nose, eye, and jaw. I've diagnosed this horrible condition a few times, and the characteristic symptom is deep ear pain that can be triggered by touching the ear canal.

Initially, the pain is sharp and shooting, then it subsides to a dull ache. Unfortunately, geniculate neuralgia may be misdiagnosed as a TMJ problem, especially if the sufferer also has clicking or popping in the TMJ. I treated one patient who developed this problem after TMJ surgery.

Aneurysms, adendocystic carcinoma of the ear canal, or (most commonly), a blood vessel malformation can cause geniculate neuralgia.

Geniculate neuralgia is treated with medication (Tegretal, Baclofen or Neurontin) and topical anesthetics. Some cases respond well to microvascular decompression surgery, a neurosurgical technique primarily used to treat trigeminal neuralgia.

Bell's Palsy

You wake up one morning and one side of your face feels very strange. You can't smile, close your eye, or pucker your lips. There's generally little pain, but certainly you're very alarmed. This sudden paralysis of the muscles on one side of your face is called Bell's Palsy.

The most common disorder of the facial nerve, Bell's palsy is most likely caused by a viral infection (probably, the herpes simplex virus) within the ear, producing swelling on the facial nerve as it exits the skull and runs through the temporal bone near the ear. This facial paralysis seems to also be caused by trauma to the face. In rare cases, Bell's palsy may be caused by a tumor in the temporal bone of the skull.

The facial nerve, or seventh cranial nerve, resembles a telephone cable because it contains as many as 7,000 individual nerve fibers. Each fiber has the potential to carry the electrical impulses to specific facial muscles (called, muscles of facial expression) which permits us to smile, frown, or make any number of facial expressions. When approximately half or more of these nerve fibers are interrupted (usually by swelling around the nerve), the facial muscles sag or are paralyzed.

The facial nerve also carries fibers which provide taste sensation to the front 2/3 of the tongue. So, if you suffer with Bell's palsy, it's quite possible you'll have temporary loss of some of your taste in addition to facial paralysis.

Bell's palsy effects approximately 40,000 Americans each year. It can strike anyone at any age, but it disproportionately attacks pregnant women, those who have diabetes, the flu or cold, or other types of upper respiratory illnesses.

In addition to one-sided facial paralysis, other symptoms of Bell's palsy may include pain, drooling, tearing, and hyper-sensitivity to sounds.

Immediate treatment is very important! If you're not treated immediately--within two weeks--you have a 20% chance of having one side of your face paralyzed forever. However, if treated quickly, you reduce your chances or permanent damage tremendously.

There's no set way to treat Bell's palsy. However, generally we use cortisone to reduce inflammation, anti-viral drugs (e.g., Acyclovir 400 mg 5 times/day), and an eye patch to protect the eye from drying at nighttime. During the day, we prescribe artificial tears to keep the eye moist and, sometimes, a clear eye patch. Non-conventional therapies like acupuncture, massage therapy, and acupressure are known to help some patients.

If you're involved in contact sports (like karate), and if you've suffered with Bell's palsy, wear head protection to protect your facial nerves.

Patients with permanent facial paralysis may be rehabilitated through a variety of surgical procedures including eyelid weights or springs, muscle transplants, and nerve stimulators. Other treatments include a special form of physical therapy and, at times, chemical injections (called botox injections) to weaken over-active muscles. Consult an ENT physician concerning Bell's palsy.

Chapter Summary

Craniofacial pain disorders are rarely recognized and worse, often misdiagnosed and mistreated. The face and its deeper structures are highly innervated, and when a structure is injured, pain is frequently referred to other areas of the face, head, and neck.

Consult dentists trained in the diagnosis and treatment of these pain disorders. Don't allow anyone to perform surgery until the source of the pain is successfully identified. If you feel uneasy about a suggested procedure, get a second or even third opinion.

Due to the anatomical complexity of the face and head, a proper diagnosis is difficult, at times, to find. This is the most challenging aspect of my job. Most of us can mentally and physically deal with leg or arm pain, but facial pain commands our complete attention.

Lastly, realize that more than one of these (and other) disorders may occur together. That's why you need to consult a doctor trained in craniofacial and temporomandibular joint disorders.

References

1. *Insight Into Facial Nerve Problems.* American Academy of Otolaryngology–Head and Neck Surgery. Alexandria, Virginia, 1997.

2. **Shankland WE:** *Craniofacial pain syndromes that mimic temporomandibular joint disorders.* Ann Acad Med (Singapore) 1995;24:83-112.

CHAPTER Nine

Sinusitis

What's the most frequent problem portrayed in television advertisements? Sinus problems! You'd think everyone suffered from sinusitis. Unfortunately, many doctors also believe this.

According to the standard classification of headaches, pain from sinus inflammation accounts for only 2% or so of all headaches, although sinusitis may affect an estimated 14 percent of the population, according to a report published in the June 1998, issue of the *Journal of Allergy and Clinical Immunology*. In my practice, patients and doctors blame sinusitis and migraines for nearly all head pain. It just "ain't" so.

We have four different types of paranasal (along side of the nose) sinuses, any or all of which can become inflamed, causing headache and facial pain. They are located on either side of the nose (maxillary sinuses), behind and in between the eyes (ethmoid sinuses), in the forehead (frontal sinuses), and further back in the head (sphenoid sinuses) in the skull base. All four are paired, meaning there's a right and left sinus. The ethmoidal sinuses are actually many small (3 to 15 on each side) air-filled chambers within the ethmoid bones. They were created to reduce the weight of the skull and provide voice resonance.

> *We have four different types of paranasal (along side of the nose) sinuses, any or all of which can become inflamed, causing headache and facial pain.*

The trigeminal nerve provides the nerve supply to all these sinuses, as well as the nose. That's why any sinus inflammation may refer pain to the eyes, teeth, jaws, TMJ, neck and even the back of the head and why sinus problems are frequently confused with other medical conditions.

The autonomic nervous system, which travels with trigeminal branches, controls normal sinus functions, causing the blood vessels in the linings of the sinuses to engorge with blood, activating one set of sinuses to function for a while and then, almost on cue, the blood vessels in the sinuses on the other side engorge. This engorgement warms air passing through the sinuses and exposes certain white blood cells, created to fight bacteria, to function and protect the rest of our body. Have you ever noticed a feeling of pressure release in one side of your nose? That's when the autonomic nervous system produced the engorging of the other side.

All sinuses are air-containing cavities that develop as extensions of the nasal passages. They're lined with the same type of thin, mucous membrane as the nose. This lining secretes mucous, traps particles in air we breathe, and warms the incoming air. Also, these sinuses are lined with a type of cell which produces tiny hair-like projections termed cilia.

For sinuses to function properly, air must pass over these mucous membranes. Containing bacteria, dirt, pollen, and pollutants, mucous is moved by the cilia towards specific ostia (Latin for doors or entrances and anatomically, a short hairpin-shaped tube) or openings into the nasal cavities. Each ostium is only about 1/6 of an inch in diameter and is easily blocked. Any changes that cause blockage of these ostia produce an environment for sinusitis to develop. You can feel the pressure build up while the ostia are closed. Unfortunately, these holes or ostia are located at the top of the sinus, making drainage difficult.

Sinusitis, the inflammation of one or more of these sinuses, may be acute or chronic (lasting longer than three months). Acute sinusitis most often causes facial pain, while headaches from sinusitis are generally due to a chronic problem. Sinusitis starts with the blockage of the ostium of the sinuses. When this occurs, mucus that normally is expelled from the sinus into the nose builds up in the sinus. This can cause pressure, pain, or both.

Mucus is also an excellent breading ground for bacteria. If mucus is not cleared from the sinus immediately through the ostia, an abscess can develop in the sinus. An abscess is a pus-pocket inside a closed space.

Allergies, upper respiratory infections, and small particles produce inflammation, which in turn, causes a thickening of the mucous membranes. The swelling of the mucous membranes closes the ostia, preventing the normal flow of mucous out of the sinus into the nasal cavity. This closing off of the sinus or sinuses is the underlying mechanical cause for sinusitis.

Diagnosis. How is sinusitis diagnosed? It's difficult to diagnose a sinus infection early in the course of the disease. After taking a careful history and doing a physical exam, the diagnosis is made by looking inside the nose with a flexible rubber or rigid steel tube called an endoscope. Depending on what's found with endoscopy, an x-ray and CT scan of the sinuses may be ordered. Don't worry about endoscopy. Your nose is first sprayed with a local anesthetic.

If you suspect you have sinusitis, why not take this short quiz, courtesy of the American Academy of Otolaryngology-Head and Neck Surgery? See if you have any of the following:

- Facial pain or pressure ___Yes ___No
- Headache ___ Yes ___ No
- Congestion or stuffy nose ___ Yes ___ No
- Post-nasal drip ___ Yes ___ No
- Thick, yellow-green discharge . ___ Yes ___ No
- Cold symptoms more than 10 days ___ Yes ___ No
- Low grade fever ___ Yes ___ No
- Bad Breath ___ Yes ___ No
- Pain in upper back teeth ___ Yes ___ No

A score of three "Yes" answers or more may indicate that you have sinusitis and you need to see your physician.

Treatment. There are many forms of treatment of sinusitis. Commonly used antibiotics such as penicillin, erythromycin, and tetracycline don't generally work because often the bacteria are resistant. Antibiotics such as amoxicillin and sulfa drugs may be used first for sinus infections, but they don't work in patients who've had infections for any length of time or who've previously taken multiple antibiotics, probably because bacteria frequently develop resistance to antibiotics. In that case, a newer antibiotic is needed. Unfortunately, they're expensive, sometimes costing $100 per week or more.

Although antibiotics are essential in treating sinus infections, it's just as critical to aid the mucus in the sinuses to drain adequately. Nasal sprays, containing small amounts of cortisone to reduce the inflammation inside the nose and around the ostia, can be helpful.

We also use over-the-counter decongestants like Sudafed to reduce the swelling inside the nose. Prescription medications such as Guaifenesin (the active ingredient in Robitussin) effectively reduce the thickness of the mucus trapped within the sinuses. They are needed in high dosages, typically 2400 mg. per day. The most common effects are thirst and drowsiness.

Can you use an over-the-counter nasal spray? *Very judiciously.* Decongestant nasal sprays, such as Neosynephrine or Vicks Sinex can be used according to directions for three to seven days but no longer. Use extreme caution in order to prevent worsening of symptoms or addiction to these sprays.

Consider using a vaporizer. Hot mist vaporizers work best. Place the vaporizer beside your bed every night. The moisture will help thin out the mucus. Also, breathe in the steam of moist vapor on a regular basis by boiling water, though this isn't as effective as a vaporizer. High humidity is best, but for those suffering also with allergies to molds and dust mites, keep the humidity less than 50%. Purchase a humidity gauge from a hardware store.

Can antihistamines treat sinusitis? Under rare circumstances, but only if allergies play a prominent part in the symptoms. Because antihistamines dry mucous membranes, we avoid them when treating sinusitis. The mucus in the sinuses may then be dried out and plastered up against the wall of the sinuses. The bacteria grow well because they're trapped inside the sinuses and then can't be moved out. At first, people feel better because the volume of mucous in the sinuses is initially reduced, but eventually symptoms return.

It's important to drink a minimum of eight, 8 ounce glasses of water per day. Ideally, 15 or 20 glasses is helpful in order to thin the mucus out and allow adequate drainage.

Can you drink alcohol when you have a sinus infection? Alcohol causes worsening of sinusitis, and it's a diuretic, causing your kidneys to remove more water than necessary from your blood. You may become dehydrated, leading to drying and thickening of the mucus. This adds to the blockage of the opening of the sinuses and a worsening of the infection.

Avoid airborne irritants. Auto exhaust, gasoline fumes, paint fumes, perfume, roach spray and household chemicals such as bleach, and cigarette smoke paralyze the tiny hairs (cilia), which move mucus out of the sinuses. These also cause irritation and inflammation in the nose and respiratory tract. There's no good way to effectively treat these exposures, so avoid them. Air filters help, especially HEPA filters, the most efficient of air filters.

And surgery? A small percentage of patients with chronic sinusitis fail to improve with the best medical treatment, usually less than 10%. Surgery is frequently performed on patients who haven't had the best medical treatment prior to surgery. Always get a second opinion.

Maxillary Sinusitis.

The most common type of sinusitis, maxillary sinusitis, is often blamed for mid-facial, upper jaw, or headache pain. The maxillary

The most common type of sinusitis, maxillary sinusitis, is often blamed for mid-facial, upper jaw, or headache pain.

sinus is shaped like a pyramid and is located in the back of our upper jaws, above the molars.

Acute Maxillary Sinusitis. Generally, acute maxillary sinusitis develops as a direct extension of a nose or tooth infection. Especially in those who have lost some of their upper posterior teeth because the roots of the remaining upper back teeth often extend through the floor of the maxillary sinus. Often, after a tooth is treated with a root canal or removed, an infection of the lining of the sinus occurs. In fact, maxillary sinusitis occurs about 15% of the time after a tooth is removed, infected or not.

Whether it's an allergy, an infected tooth, or an upper respiratory infection, if the lining of the maxillary sinus thickens as a response, the flow of mucous is slowed or stopped, the sinus can't drain, and sinusitis develops.

The most common symptoms of acute maxillary sinusitis are:

- Headaches in the forehead
- Pain and tenderness over the cheek
- Mid-facial pain which radiates into the ear
- Nose bleeding
- Generalized feeling of tiredness or feeling run-down
- A low grade fever
- Upper back tooth pain, especially when chewing
- Nasal or post-nasal drainage
- An unpleasant taste or smell
- Numbness in the roof of the mouth (at times)

All the above symptoms worsen if you bend over. Most of these symptoms must be present if someone is suffering with acute maxillary sinusitis. Can't you see that most people who think they have sinusitis really don't? Acute sinusitis makes a person very ill.

Chronic Maxillary Sinusitis. It seems odd, but often, people suffering with chronic maxillary sinusitis have no pain. They usually complain of a runny nose, post-nasal drip, and feel blockage or pressure in the cheek.

If both maxillary sinuses are affected, the person may suffer from a diffuse headache which may be dull usually, but at other times, severe, often misdiagnosed as cluster headaches.

X-rays, CT scans, or an MRI will quickly show if the maxillary sinus is the source of pain. Like acute maxillary sinusitis, there's tenderness in the cheek. Some doctors also use a couple of blood tests (e.g., C-reactive protein and erythrocyte sedimentation rate).

Ethmoid Sinusitis

Located in the upper back of the nose, the ethmoid sinuses (or air cells) are likened to 8 or 10 balloons placed in an oblong box and inflated. Each air cell opens into the nasal cavity so that mucous drains into the nose. Each air cell varies in size and shape and is connected to the others.

Acute Ethmoid Sinusitis. This type of sinusitis is the most common acute kind and is usually preceded by a viral upper respiratory infection. It's the only type of sinusitis which affects infants, because the ethmoid sinuses are the first to develop.

Symptoms include:

- Forehead and eye pain
- Reduced smell and taste
- Postnasal drainage
- Swelling of the skin over the eyes and upper nose
- Fever
- Runny nose
- Positive x-ray findings

This type of sinusitis is difficult to treat and is often resistant to antibiotics, probably due to the scant blood supply to the ethmoid sinuses. Antibiotics and gentle suction are helpful treatments.

Chronic Ethmoid Sinusitis. Chronic nasal infections and the development of polyps (over-growth of the mucous membrane) characterize chronic ethmoid sinusitis. These patients generally complain of dull, episodic headaches located between or behind the eyes and in the forehead area.

Fortunately, chronic ethmoid sinusitis responds well to antibiotic therapy.

Frontal Sinusitis

The frontal sinuses are located above the eyes. They're connected to the nasal fossa (nasal cavity) of the same side by the nasofrontal duct.

Acute Frontal Sinusitis. Acute frontal sinusitis is caused by any process that interferes with the normal drainage of the sinus through the nasofrontal duct. This blockage is usually pathological (i.e., an infection), but it may also be anatomical.

Head trauma can cause acute frontal sinusitis, producing swelling of the mucous membranes. Swimming, sudden exposure to high altitudes, or infections arising in the maxillary sinus can also cause acute frontal sinusitis.

Symptoms of acute frontal sinusitis include:

- Pain in the forehead which begins about an hour after rising and peaks around noon

- Generalized headache that can include the temples, top or even back of the head

- Head pain that's intensified by bending over or tapping on the forehead

- Fever

Acute frontal sinusitis can be dangerous because either a brain abscess or osteomyelitis (bone inflammation) of the frontal bone may form. Intravenous antibiotics, bed rest, and topical medications are usually effective treatments. If rapid improvement fails to occur, surgical drainage is usually recommended.

Chronic Frontal Sinusitis. Unlike most chronic sinusitis, chronic frontal sinusitis is painful, and usually generates dull and constant headache accompanied with pressure. This is a serious condition and demands aggressive medical intervention.

Sphenoid Sinusitis

Located within the sphenoid bone in the base of the skull, there are two sphenoidal sinuses: a right and left. With a partition between, they're rarely symmetrical. Like all the other paranasal sinuses, the trigeminal nerve supplies somatosensory (feeling) to sphenoidal sinuses, and the parasympathetic nervous system controls the functions of the mucous membrane lining. Sphenoid sinusitis is the least common form of sinusitis and is usually associated with ethmoid sinusitis.

Acute Sphenoid Sinusitis. Frequently caused by such activities as deep sea diving, head trauma, cocaine sniffing, and radiation of the head, acute sphenoid sinusitis also tends to afflict people with diabetes, leukemia, and immunosuppression (e.g., AIDS).

Rarely is sphenoid sinusitis the primary cause of headache or facial pain. However, an acutely infected sphenoid sinus can cause:

- Forehead, temporal, mastoid, and occipital headaches
- Pain behind the eyes
- Dizziness
- Fever
- Postnasal drainage
- Sleeplessness
- Mental symptoms
  (e.g., forgetfulness, lack of concentration)
- Positive x-ray findings

As with other types of sinusitis, we treat acute sphenoid sinusitis with decongestants, rest, antibiotics, pain medication, and the application of heat to the painful area of the head or face. If symptoms continue, surgery is considered.

Chronic Sphenoid Sinusitis. This is a very rare condition, but when present is often mis-diagnosed as atypical facial pain, trigeminal neuralgia, brain tumor, migraine headache, or carotid artery aneurysm (or, a weakened area in the wall of an artery). Polyps may develop.

Various types of surgical treatment are used to treat chronic sphenoid sinusitis. Fortunately, since the advent of antibiotics, sphenoid sinusitis rarely develops.

Chapter Summary _____

Sinusitis is a common and painful disorder. Because many patients and doctors use the term sinusitis for any type of facial and undiagnosed head pain, sinusitis is often a waste basket diagnosis.

Aside from facial or head pain, fever, tiredness and sickness characterize sinusitis. Fever is the important symptom, as many other orofacial pain syndromes do not produce an increase in body temperature.

Avoid using nasal sprays to self-treat yourself for longer than a few days if you suspect you're suffering from sinusitis. Although helpful for short durations, nasal sprays may cause severe complications, possibly even worse than the symptoms of sinusitis.

Obtain a second opinion if a doctor suggests surgical treatment. I've seen too many patients still suffering after sinus surgery. The number of people who have submitted to multiple sinus surgeries, only to continue with facial or head pain, embarrasses the medical profession.

The normal, anatomical conditions of the paranasal sinuses (e.g., moist, dark environment) make all of us susceptible to sinus infections. See your doctor rather than diagnosing and treating yourself.

CHAPTER Ten

Fibromyalgia, Myofascial Pain Syndrome and Orofacial Pain

With Devin Starlanyl, M.D.

What's Fibromyalgia?

Fibromyalgia syndrome (FMS) is a non-degenerative, non-inflammatory chronic pain syndrome that affects the musculoskeletal (muscles and skeleton) system. It's characterized by fatigue, non-restorative sleep (poor sleep), morning muscle stiffness, and specific muscle tender points. FMS isn't a term describing only achy muscles. It's not that simple, and that's why there's so much confusion and misinformation about it among sufferers and doctors.

> *Fibromyalgia characterized by fatigue, non-restorative sleep (poor sleep), morning muscle stiffness, and specific muscle tender points.*

These tender points hurt when you press them, but they don't refer pain elsewhere. A common test used by physicians, the "eleven out of eighteen tender points" used to identify FMS patients, was clearly meant to establish criteria for research studies, and was never intended for clinical applications. FMS is actually a biochemical dis-regulation of the metabolic and neuroendocrine (nervous control of glands) systems.

The fact that FMS is biochemical means you can't have fibromyalgia only of the back, shoulders, or neck. If you have it, you have it all over. It causes a generalized deep tissue ache, like a flu that never ends.

Think of a person with fibromyalgia as a stereo system stuck with its volume turned up. Your sensations amplify and sometimes change. Noises may seem so loud they hurt. The same may be true for light, smells and touch. At times, your taste is also different. FMS intensifies pain perception. These nervous system changes are termed plasticity, which means the normal settings of the nervous system are changed.

FMS intensifies pain perception.

Healing and regulatory processes of the body take place during deep, delta-level sleep. With FMS, delta sleep patterns in the brain are often interrupted by alpha (waking) waves. Whenever you reach deep sleep, it's interrupted, sending you into shallow sleep or worse, into a wakeful state. In the morning, you get out of bed worn out, sometimes feeling worse than you did when you went to sleep.

It isn't enough you spend eight hours in bed. You need to wake up feeling as though you have slept, so that you can fully function. This doesn't happen when delta sleep is interrupted. So, if you have a TMJ or orofacial pain problem or need routine dental treatment, you might experience more pain and may take longer to heal.

You can do a lot for FMS. For example, the chronic fatigue of FMS often disappears once you regain restorative sleep. FMS isn't progressive. If it worsens, that indicates the perpetuating factors, such as non-restorative sleep, are not being properly addressed or a co-existing condition, such as myofascial pain syndrome (MPS), is developing. It's important you that and your medical care provider understand the differences between FMS and MPS.

What Is Myofascial Pain Syndrome?

Myofascial pain syndrome (MPS) is a neuromuscular condition characterized with nodules and ropey bands of trigger points (TrPs) that not only hurt, but also cause muscular weakness, decreased range of motion, autonomic nervous system symptoms, and referred pain. A trigger point is an area that's tender when pressed, but it also triggers (in the sense of activating) a referred pain pattern elsewhere in the body. Localized pain is often mistakenly called FMS. This is confusing because some of the tender points of FMS are common MPS TrP sites, but remember, FMS tender areas don't refer pain when pressed.

Each myofascial TrP has a specific referral area that causes pain and other symptoms such as autonomic referred symptoms, which are symptoms other than pain, such as dizziness, alteration of perceptions of light and dark patterns, weight, and spatial location. These confuse you and your doctor.

> *Some of the tender points of FMS are common MPS trigger point sites, but remember, FMS tender areas don't refer pain when pressed.*

Sleep disturbances are also common, due to pain from TrPs. Like FMS, MPS isn't progressive. If it seems progressive, it's because trigger points are developing satellite and secondary TrPs due to failure to address adequately the perpetuating factors (e.g., over-exertion, sitting under a cold air duct, stress, performing work or exercise without properly warming up, and trauma). When TrPs develop throughout the body, the referral patterns overlap, which makes it harder to separate the individual TrPs, and more difficult to distinguish MPS from FMS. Fibromyalgia and myofascial pain due to TrPs are two of the most common pain syndromes, yet they require different treatments.

These conditions must be recognized as separate conditions before an effective treatment strategy can be planned. Physicians must be thoroughly familiar with TrP referral patterns in order to recognize the source of the symptoms. It's not uncommon for the MPS trigger points to be the pain initiator, and the FMS to be the pain amplifier. For physicians to understand adequately the magnitude of the pain experienced by what we call the FMS & MPS Complex, they need to understand the individual components.

Pain is a major perpetuating factor, and until the pain is adequately treated, the patient has little chance of improvement. The key in both FMS and MPS is always to identify the perpetuating factors, and deal with them thoroughly.

Informational Substances

To understand the nature of fibromyalgia and how it affects orofacial pain, you need to know a little about informational substances, neurotransmitters, peptides, and other biochemicals that regulate body processes. Many informational substances are regulated during delta level sleep. We're just beginning to learn about informational substances.

The neuron, or nerve cell, is highly specialized. It notices changes in its environment, and sends information about these changes to other neurons by releasing an electrochemical called a neurotransmitter. Messages travel to the brain from neuron to neuron by a series of neurotransmitter transfers.

Neurotransmitters exist for only a brief time. Once released by a neuron, the neurotransmitter travels across a small space between neurons (the synapse) and stimulates the next neuron to react. Then the neurotransmitter is broken down, and the chemical components are absorbed by the body. Many neurotransmitters work in pairs, forming a balance. One will produce an effect, and the other will stop that effect. This balance keeps a single neurotransmitter from going out of control.

In FMS, this regulating system breaks down, and these vitally important balances are lost. Each informational substance has many functions to perform. Listed on page 45 are a few substances which function as neurotransmitters. How they influence orofacial pain syndromes is discussed.

Histamine. Histamine is the substance often associated with allergies. When your cell membranes are broken by trauma, such as a bruise or cut, or exposed to heat or chemical toxins, histamine is released. Histamine causes the smooth muscle of the bronchial area to constrict, so we become short of breath. It relaxes small blood vessels, but constricts large ones. Histamine provokes a generalized dilation of the blood vessels in parts of the brain, as any of us who have ever had a "histamine headache" know very well.

Histamine also causes an increase in the permeability (physiological leaking) of the capillaries. Swelling results as intracellular components leak into the area outside the cells. When histamine levels become high, swelling and a runny nose occur. This congestion adds misery to orofacial pain.

Acetylcholine. In those afflicted with FMS, an increase in acetylcholine increases the amount of mucus in the upper respiratory tract. Acetylcholine is also involved with speech and sensory processes. It adds to the general confusion that pain brings and amplifies pain and swelling.

Noradrenaline and adrenaline. These two chemicals, noradrenaline (norepinephrine) and adrenaline (epinephrine) are very similar and are associated with energy consumption. Adrenaline, released during stressful episodes, initiates a complex series of reactions throughout the body. Muscles tighten. Respiration rates increase. Small blood vessels constrict. The adrenaline stress reaction enhances our consciousness of pain, which again increases our sensitivity to pain.

When noradrenaline is released, the hypothalamus directs the body to lower its temperature, and the thalamus lowers the pain threshold. Noradrenaline increases our perception of pain, creates anxiety that contributes to the apprehension of pain, and adds to the overall stress reaction.

Serotonin. Serotonin influences sleep, moods, and vomiting and is another biochemical that affects those with FMS. Levels of this neurotransmitter are controlled by the balance of adrenaline and noradrenaline. Serotonin also affects the balance of the pain threshold.

If you have a migraine attack, serotonin plays a role, causing constriction of all major blood vessels in the head. Serotonin may produce visual disturbances classic to migraines by constricting retinal blood vessels. This may be part of the reason why some of us see "stars" when we cough. Following such constriction, the blood vessels dilate, resulting in a throbbing headache and nausea.

Substance P. Substance P is an informational substance that functions as a local neurotransmitter, influencing the balance between the hypothalamus, pituitary, and adrenal glands, called the HPA axis. Substance P regulates sensory mechanisms, causes constriction in the airways, and may increase mucus production, increasing congestion.

It's important to know that having FMS doesn't mean a lack of neurotransmitters. Some with FMS have high levels of some neurotransmitters and low levels of others. For example, there may be too much histamine and too little serotonin or others neurotransmitters. There are many factions or subsets of fibromyalgia. No two patients are alike. In addition, the levels of neurotransmitters vary hour by hour and day by day. That's one more reason why FMS patients so frustrate doctors. Each sufferer requires specific care.

The HPA-Axis

In fibromyalgia, there's a disrupted HPA axis. In other words, the critical balance among the hypothalamus, pituitary gland, and adrenal glands is no longer operating properly. The balance among the hormones of these glands is an important key to the proper functioning of the body.

A small gland located deep within the brain, the hypothalamus is the body's thermostat. When we're in danger, it signals its neighbor, the pituitary gland, to prepare the body to react. Then, the pituitary gland sends a chemical message through the blood to the adrenal glands, which are a pair of tiny glands perched on top of the kidneys. These minuscule but mighty glands influence almost all of the body's systems by producing adrenaline and many other biochemicals the body uses in stressful situations. All of these glands communicate by neurotransmitters.

What the relationship between the HPA axis and fibromyalgia? According to Dr. Ronald Melzack, one of the world's leading neuroscientists in pain research, chronic stress (both physical and emotional), causes a disruption in the body's homeostasis (normal body functions producing health) and thus over-activity of the HPA axis can cause fibromyalgia and many other chronic pain syndromes.

Hormones

Secreted by glands, hormones are specialized biochemicals dependant on each other. Connected by chemical feedback loops, they help to regulate the production of a specific hormone. This regulation often fails in FMS, because hormones are also influenced by neurotransmitters.

The effects of hormones last much longer than neurotransmitters because hormones aren't broken down immediately after being used. Unlike neurotransmitters, which are released, travel a short distance, and are then broken down, hormones are released into the circulatory system and travel vast distances to perform their designated functions. They exist from the time they're released from a gland or specialized cell, during their circulation through the body, until they arrive at their specific receptors elsewhere in the body.

Other hormones act on the cells near their release point. Dysfunctional neurotransmitters often lead to dysfunctional hormones. Surely, aren't we "fearfully and wonderfully" made? (Psalm 139:12-14)

Muscles

There are two basic types of muscle: smooth and striated (skeletal). Smooth muscles function automatically, independent of consciousness. They're under the direction of the autonomic nervous system. Autonomic sounds like automatic and, in this case, it is.

By contrast, a striated muscle is the type we usually think of when we think of a muscle. We voluntarily contract them to move our bodies. But, the autonomic nervous system also tells striated muscles to function without our knowledge. We tense these muscles involuntarily to prepare to fight or to flee danger. When the danger's over, the autonomic nervous system commands our skeletal muscles to relax . . . usually.

Unfortunately, with FMS, the autonomic nervous system often malfunctions, forgetting to command the skeletal muscles to relax. If the skeletal muscles don't relax but remain constricted (that is, stay tightly contracted), they continue to react to a stressful situation that's no longer present. Imagine what happens then? That's right . . . the development of trigger points and muscle pain.

> *Unfortunately, with FMS, the autonomic nervous system often malfunctions, forgetting to command the skeletal muscles to relax.*

Muscles were created to contract, function and then relax. Keep them warm and well stretched, including your facial muscles. If you're restricting your mouth movements while chewing and opening your mouth, ask your dentist for some exercises.

Don't forget to stretch your eye muscles. Tight eye muscles can cause pain in the surrounding areas of the head and face. This is especially true if you have both FMS and MPS. Put one hand on your head, above your forehead, and try to look at your hand. This shouldn't hurt. If it does, the TrPs in your muscles are telling you they're present. With your eyes still looking upward at your hand, look from one upper corner of your eye to the other. If this hurts, the TrPs are there too, and that's at least part of what is causing your eye problems.

The eye exercises will help stretch-out eye muscle TrPs. You must do them regularly to prevent the TrPs from recurring. Their tightness makes orofacial pain far worse.

Symptoms Adding to Orofacial Pain

Teeth clenching is a default mechanism of the brain. With mixed or erratic signals, you clench your jaw–a sort of twiddling of the cranial thumbs. This happens a lot with FMS. There are special medications and oral appliances to help manage clenching. Discuss this problem with your doctors.

At times, many FMS patients have vasomotor rhinitis. That's a runny nose with no infectious or allergic cause. With muscle tightening, normal fluid passages are constricted, and fluid backs up in the sinuses. This fluid can be considerable, thanks to our dysfunctional neurotransmitters. So we get a constant postnasal drip all night, although the membranes of the nose may feel dry and even bleed. This dryness becomes severe if you live in air conditioned spaces, cold areas, or use a wood stove. If your nasal secretions get thick and won't flow, ask your doctor about the medication Guaifenesin.

Be sure to look into the reason behind the post nasal drip. If it continues, it can lead to a mechanical sore throat, which is an invitation to infection. FMS & MPS nocturnal sinus syndrome is a nighttime sinus stuffiness that occurs on one side of the head. Gravity drains the congestion to the lower side, so the stuffy side moves as you toss and turn in the night. This condition accompanies postnasal drip and a constantly runny nose.

Trigger points form from this irritation, which eventually refers pain to the upper back teeth. You've probably noticed that at times when you use a hot washcloth on your face, your nose starts running. Before going to bed, use hot moist compresses on your cheeks and along the sides of your nose. Try to loosen some of the congestion. Use warm salt water as nose drops to help prevent nighttime sinus congestion.

The inside of your mouth can become very fragile with FMS. This can worsen during the menstrual period, or at other times that your immune and other body systems are stressed. You may experience sores, bumps inside the mouth, and bleeding gums. Your cheek lining may tear from eating a piece of toast.

It isn't unusual for people with FMS and other chronic illnesses to have a viral disease, especially Herpes Simplex Type 1, as a perpetuating factor. Cold sores, canker sores, and aphthous mouth ulcers may develop. Crops of isolated pimples, filled with clear fluid, may appear on the skin. They can change to eczema-like patches, which may remain for weeks. Check for a folic acid deficiency.

Oral niacinamide or Lactinex, Zovirax or Aphthsol ointment may help. If you're having an outbreak and have a dental visit scheduled, discuss this with your dentist.

Dental Treatment

Many FMS patients can't tolerate epinephrine in some of the local anesthetics used by dentists. If you can't sleep or experience a FMS "flare up" after local anesthesia, talk to your dentist. Unfortunately, the doctor may have no any idea what you're talking about, so try to educate him about FMS and MPS. If you have co-existing myofascial TrPs, take frequent rests to exercise your mouth during dental visits. This is especially needed for prolonged procedures like routine cleanings, multiple restorations (fillings), or crown preparation.

It's not unusual for people with both myofascial TrPs and FMS to experience sore ridges in the area of their cheeks that run parallel to the tops of the lower molars. If fact, this line (linea alba or white line in Latin) is normal. But for those with MPS or FMS, the linea alba in both cheeks often enlarge. We've had many patients terrified they had oral cancer when the problem simply was FMS and exaggerated linea alba.

You may have a problem knowing where your teeth are in relation to your body. You bite your cheek, lips or tongue, adding to your stress load. When this happens, apply warm compresses over your face, but be cautious not to burn your skin. The problem with jaw proprioception (knowing where your jaw is in space) is characteristic of FMS and MPS. Slow down when chewing or talking.

People with FMS & MPS also have more difficulty adjusting to dentures, probably due to the FMS amplification of pain and distortion in proprioception of the muscles of mastication (the muscles that move the jaw) while chewing. It's important that dental problems be fixed promptly. A denture wearer often returns to the dentist many times for denture adjustments–far more than those who don't suffer with FMS or MPS. Any imbalances in the occlusion (bite) must be corrected, particularly when the patient is relaxed and his muscles aren't painful. If they aren't, sore spots, headaches, and orofacial pain develop.

FMS and MPS patients with new restorations also return frequently to the dentist for adjustments to the occlusion. This frustrates both the patient and doctor. The muscles which move the jaw actually are fighting your normal jaw position, and this makes the intricate procedure of occlusal adjustment very difficult. As with occlusal problems with dentures, headaches, ear and TMJ pain, and orofacial pain may develop. Teeth also become sensitive and even mobile. Far too many teeth are treated with root canals and ultimately, removed simply because the occlusion needs refining. These problems are magnified with FMS and MPS. Angry patients go to another dentist only to have the same problems. Have patience with your doctor.

Therapy

There are many therapies for FMS and MPS. Initially, you may be able to tolerate nothing more than moist heat, passive stretching, and medications. Because bodywork (physical therapy techniques) promotes the release of trapped toxins and wastes, fatigue and nausea may arise. These symptoms indicate you must go slowly.

Just as with MPS, the FMS sufferer must identify perpetuating factors, such as lack of restorative sleep. The body needs time to detoxify with gentle, brief, and non-repetitive stretching (when tolerated). At first, bodywork may not be tolerable more than once a week. Once you regain restorative sleep, healing proceeds much faster with adequate pain control and a proper diet. No cure exits yet for fibromyalgia, but a lot of researchers are working on it. You can improve the quality of your life, even if you have both FMS and MPS. There's a lot of hope for an even brighter tomorrow.

Thanks to Dr. Paul St. Amand, we now have an effective way to treat FMS. He discovered that a common medication, *Guaifenesin*, worked extremely well in reducing the symptoms of fibromyalgia. We've followed Dr. St. Amand's recommended therapy and have witnessed dramatic improvement of the symptoms of FMS. Unfortunately, most doctors and pharmacists haven't heard of this therapy yet.

Surgical Therapy? Recently, a few neurosurgeons have been experimentally treating fibromyalgia with surgery. Apparently, this radical procedure has helped some patients by removing bone at the base of the skull to eliminate compression on the lower part of the brain and upper spinal cord. By removing bone in certain areas to enlarge the space for these vital tissues, any inappropriate pressure on the pathway for all the nervous system from the brain to the rest of the body is stopped. In theory, for some sufferers of FMS, this reduction of pressure cures their symptoms.

I'm certainly not endorsing or even suggesting this dangerous procedure, especially as a first choice. It appears to help only those with abnormal MRI findings (Chiari malformations) at the base of the brain, where a portion of the cerebellum protrudes through the foramen magnum, the opening at the base of the skull. But most FMS patients have no abnormal neurological findings. In fact, we believe most fibromyalgia symptoms are due to neurotransmitter problems, a disruption of the HPA axis, but not a physical impingement on nervous tissues.

Be cautious. Before you jump to inappropriate conclusions, consider the following:

- The operations should be considered only for patients with abnormal neurological exams and abnormal findings on MRIs of the base of the skull and neck. Unfortunately, most FMS patients are never examined neurologically.

- This surgical treatment must definitely be considered experimental. It's too early to tell how long results will last and which patients might most benefit. The results from these neurosurgeons need to be published and examined by others. That has not yet happened.

- Although preliminary reports suggest that about 50% of FMS patients treated surgically have seen improvement, 20% felt no improvement and 15% reported their FMS symptoms became worse. That's a large percentage.

Let's watch for any publications about long-term results of this invasive procedure. If you've had an MRI and the radiologist felt a portion of your cerebellum protrudes through the foramen magnum at the base of your skull, you may be a candidate for surgery. But get several opinions because this is a very serious and radical procedure.

References

1. **Melzack R:** *Pain and stress: a new perspective.* In, Psychosocial Factors in Pain. Gatchel RJ, Turk DC (eds). New York: The Guilford Press, 1999:89-106.

2. *Fibromyalgia & Chronic Myofascial Pain Syndrome.* **Starlanyl D,** Copeland ME. Oakland: New Harbinger Publications, 1996.

3. **Shankland WE:** *What your dentist should know.* In, The Fibromyalgia Advocate. Starlanyl DJ. Oakland: New Harbinger Publications, 1998.

4. *The Fibromyalgia Advocate.* **Starlanyl DJ.** Oakland: New Harbinger Publications, 1998.

5. *What Your Doctor May Not Tell You About Fibromyalgia.* **St. Amand RP, Marek CC.** New York: Warner Books, 1999.

Devin Starlanyl, M.D., specializes in the research and treatment of FMS and MPS. She doesn't actively treat patients at this time. Dr. Starlanyl speaks frankly as she suffers from both these conditions. Her two books (Fibromyalgia & Chronic Myofascial Pain Syndrome and The Fibromyalgia Advocate) are both best sellers and have helped thousands upon thousand of sufferers worldwide. Active in her church, Dr. Starlanyl has also written a fictional novel, Worlds of Power, Lines of Light, which has recently been released. Her web page address is: http://www.sover.net/~devstar

Eleven

Bruxism

With James Boyd, D.D.S.

Before we discuss bruxism, we should try to define this unusual term, but even the dental profession can't agree on a simple definition. Consider these comments from John Rugh, PhD, a noted authority on the subject of bruxism, "Unfortunately at this time, the exact nature of nocturnal bruxism and the mechanisms of bruxism are very poorly understood. To date, there has been no agreement on a definition of bruxism, and little is known about the biomechanics of various bruxism behaviors and how these may relate to various signs and symptoms."

Bruxism is the technical term for grinding and clenching of the teeth. These so-called parafunctional activities (para = besides or amiss, abnormal; functional = normal action or activities; therefore, parafunctional activities are abnormal activities), over a long period of time, cause abrasion of the teeth, sensitive teeth, and orofacial pain.

Dentists can tell if a patient bruxes. Usually, the tips (cusps) of the teeth are worn and look flat. As the teeth wear down and the enamel is abraded off, the inside, more organic portion of the tooth (the dentin) is exposed, causing sensitivity to cold temperatures and sweet substances. But here's the problem: Bruxism is casually defined by the objective end result of its activity (wearing of teeth), rather than by the act of parafunctional activities themselves. In other words, the dental profession diagnoses one as a bruxer because of worn, fractured teeth when the diagnosis of bruxism really should be based on the chronic contractions of the temporalis, masseter, and lateral ptergyoid muscles, the muscles chiefly responsible for moving the mandible. This diagnosis is misleading in that it focuses on the teeth, rather than on the forces generated by muscles, that effect the teeth.

For example, consider a professional football player who repeatedly injures his knee. The sports physician evaluates the injury thoroughly and asks several questions: What direction was the athlete moving? How fast was he moving? Did he make sudden stops and changes of direction? With this insight, the sports physician prescribes special therapy, exercise, and perhaps, a knee brace.

By contrast, the dentist treats the symptoms of bruxism and virtually no attempts to identify the causes are made. Only symptoms are treated, not the cause or causes. Therefore, the source of bruxism isn't addressed. In other words, we're only putting a band aide on the problem and not actually treating the problem.

Bruxism is a parafunctional activity of muscles of mastication, or the muscles which move the mandible. Parafunctional activities serve no useful purposes. Clenching of the jaws and grinding teeth are classified as parafunctional activities since food isn't chewed. The frequency, duration, and intensity of the parafunctional events dictate the patient's complaints.

Causes of Bruxism

There are many suspected causes of bruxism, but the most prevalent seems to be a correlation with sleep disturbances. Apparently, nighttime bruxers don't go through all the normal stages of sleep, remaining in the first two stages of light sleep, never progressing into deeper, more efficient and restful sleep. The lighter they sleep, the more they brux.

Other presumed causes of bruxism are:

- Emotional stress

- Caffeine

- Malocclusion (improper or bad bite)

- Alcohol

- Drugs (amphetamines, cocaine)

- Trauma to the mandible

- Genetic predisposition

- Chronic pain

- Physical exertion

Bruxism is more common than you might think. Scientists have reported that as many as 77% to 80% of people brux, but to different degrees. Interestingly, as many as 90% of bruxers are unaware of this activity. Women seem to brux more than men, but men damage their teeth more than women. On average, men exhibit the ability to clench intensely their teeth more forcibly than women.

Some researchers have reported that bruxers have a greater tendency to suffer with TMJ problems, but other researchers dispute these findings. Statistically, it's virtually impossible to prove or disprove this theory. It's unfortunate that many persons injured in motor vehicle accidents are accused of having a pre-existing TMJ problem just because they might possess evident wear patterns on their teeth, characteristic of chronic bruxing.

Whatever the causes of bruxism may be, this harmful activity is responsible for the development of many symptoms, some of which can be quite severe.

Symptoms of Bruxism

What are the signs and symptoms of bruxism? Everyone bruxes a little every time he or she sleeps, but some clench or grind their teeth hard and long, producing the following characteristic symptoms:

- Worn teeth

- Chipped teeth and broken fillings

- Jaw pain in the ear and temporomandibular joint

- Tense, painful jaw muscles

- Severe headaches

- Sensitive teeth, especially to cold temperatures

Life's stresses and certain personality types may initiate bruxism. If you're an intense person and are greatly effected by stress, then you probably brux. Such people can't relax, or worse yet, feel guilty if they try to relax. Even when sleeping, their eyes may be closed, but they toss and turn all night, and unfortunately, brux several minutes each hour. They never really rest, and they generally awaken tired and stay tired all day long.

Also, if you have a dental filling or a crown placed that changes your occlusion (bite) noticeably, you may unconsciously brux in an attempt to even-out the occlusion. You might even think you have a cavity or a fractured tooth because bruxing focuses one's attention on the first teeth to contact. This is generally the place where one bruxes the hardest.

Do I Brux?

Yes! Well, most of us do at least a few seconds each hour we sleep. But some people severely brux and don't even know it. Ask yourself the following questions:

- Do you catch yourself clenching your teeth together?

- Has anyone heard you grinding your teeth?

- Do you have frequent headaches?

- Do you often break teeth?

- Do you unconsciously place your tongue between your teeth?

- Are your jaw muscles sore, especially when waking or after eating?

- Does it hurt to chew?

- Does a tooth ever seem to get in the way when you close your mouth?

- Does it hurt to open your mouth wide?

- Do you have neck and/or shoulder pain?

- Do you awaken tired, feeling like you've never slept?

- Are your teeth sensitive to cold temperatures?

If you answered "Yes" to many of these questions, you should talk with your dentist, or ask for a referral to a dentist who treats bruxism and TMJ problems.

Anatomy of Bruxism

Two muscles are primarily responsible for bruxism: the temporalis and the lateral pterygoid. We have two of each of these muscles, one on each side of our heads. Each temporalis must work with its opposite fellow. One temporalis can't contract without the other contracting too. The temporalis, which covers the entire side of the skull, extends from behind the eye to just behind the ear. The temporalis also extends down, under the cheekbone, and attaches to the coronoid process of the mandible (Figure 11.1). The temporalis' sole task is to close and clench the jaw.

The lateral pterygoid muscle opens the mouth and moves the jaw side-to-side. Like the temporalis muscles, the lateral pterygoids work together. But unlike the temporalis, each lateral pterygoid can contract alone, pulling the jaw to the opposite side. For example, if the left one contracted, it would pull the left side of the jaw forward, which would move the jaw to the right. If both lateral pterygoids contract simultaneously, the jaw opens.

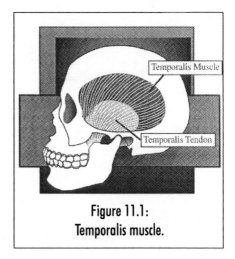

Figure 11.1:
Temporalis muscle.

Confusing matters more, understand that if the two lateral pterygoids alternately contract, the jaw swings freely side to side . . . as long as the teeth don't contact. This allows us to grind our food side to side. But when conditions are right, the lateral pterygoids also permit us to grind our teeth side-to-side.

In human beings, bruxism is a complex relationship between the temporalis' (clenching) and lateral pterygoids (grinding). Unless the teeth are brought together by the temporalis, there can be no grinding. The intensity of temporalis contraction (clenching) dictates the intensity of lateral pterygoid activity (grinding).

Bruxism, therefore, is a function of clenching. With only a slight degree of clenching, the temporalis muscles contract and, at most, only a slight amount of tooth wear occurs over a long period of time. However, as clenching intensifies (thereby, squeezing the teeth together more firmly), the contraction of the lateral pterygoids intensify, moving the jaw sideways. Consequently, if this parafunctional activity continues, teeth wear, loosening, and orofacial pain develops. Some researchers think bruxing may also damage the temporomandibular joint (TMJ), but others don't agree. These differences of opinions have been a great source of controversy in dentistry.

> *Bruxism is a function of clenching.*

Ultimately, maximal temporalis clenching prohibits all grinding movement side-to-side. The teeth don't wear -- remember, the jaw's not moving side-to-side -- even though they endure substantial amounts of force because of temporalis contraction. Maximal clenching without the influence of the lateral pterygoids protects the TMJs, yet, the temporalis muscles hurt because of chronic contraction and the development of trigger points in the muscles (tiny, consistently cramped areas in the muscle).

See how difficult it is to define bruxism? Doctors only think of intense clenching or grinding; but rarely of a combination of both parafunctional movements.

As mentioned earlier, defining bruxism is awkward. It's a complex event, and we must consider all the variations of these parafunctional jaw movements. We suggest this as a working definition of bruxism: *Intense jaw-clenching (during sleep), with or without forcible lateral jaw movements, where the intensity of clenching dictates the severity of grinding.*

Variations in symptoms depend upon a combination of the three elements of a parafunctional muscular activity associated with bruxism: (1) the frequency (number of bruxism events per night), (2) the duration of an event (how long the bruxing activity lasts), and most importantly, (3) the intensity of the contractions of the temporalis and lateral pterygoid muscles. Healthy people all have mild muscular contractions. These are easily tolerated, but highly intense bruxism activity, even for a few minutes, produces the symptoms of bruxism.

Types of Clenching

Primary Clenching. Without any opposition from the lateral pterygoids, the temporalis' contraction squeezes the jaw together in a position (called *centric relation position*) where the teeth mesh most efficiently and, ideally, permit an optimum jaw joint orientation. Regardless of the intensity of jaw clenching in this position, there's no strain on the TMJs. In fact, the jaw joints are well protected and stable. This stability allows high intensities of temporalis contractions without damaging the TMJs.

Chronic, nocturnal (nighttime) episodes of high intense temporalis contraction produces chronic myofascial pain (generalized muscle pain and tension-type headache pain when muscles in the head are involved). A recent study reported chronic tension-type headache patients (without any TMJ problem) clench their jaws while asleep, on average, **14 times more intensely than non-headache control subjects.** At one time, the term "muscle-contraction" headache was popular, but since no significant muscle contraction could be recorded during a headache event while the patient was awake, the term was changed to "tension-type" headache because it seemed like there was muscle tension.

Ongoing studies now demonstrate that nocturnal muscular parafunction is most likely the cause of tension-type headache, and quite possibly the underlying condition which allows an otherwise harmless outside influence to become a "trigger" for migraine.

Excursive Clenching. While centric clenching is the most protective to the jaw joint system, excursive (moving the jaw to the side) clenching is the most damaging. If one lateral pterygoid, say the left, were to contract, the jaw would shift to the right. Then, if the right temporalis contracted, it would squeeze a few of the right-sided teeth together, holding the jaw in an excursive position. This provides an opportunity for the left lateral pterygoid to isometrically contact, placing a continual and disruptive strain on the components of both the TMJ and the passages of the sinus walls.

Repetitive episodes often result in jaw joint damage and pain, difficulty with function, and seemingly unexplained "sinus" headaches and sinus infection. The maxillary sinus isn't really infected, but chronic excursive clenching leads patients and doctors alike to think there's an infection.

Meanwhile, the right temporalis contracts isometrically (an increase in muscle tension without changing the length of the muscle), vigorously compacting only a few teeth, whereas under normal circumstances, the forces would be distributed evenly throughout the entire dental arch. Additionally, as the left lateral pterygoid pulls the left condyle of the TMJ slightly forward, the right condyle rotates slightly, and the joint is positioned backward. Under functional circumstances (for example, chewing), this isn't a problem. However, during a prolonged isometric contraction of the temporalis in an excursive position, the many blood vessels behind the condyle are exposed to potential bruising. This scenario results in chronic headache, tender and/or painful dysfunctional jaw joints, and "phantom" toothaches (x-rays are normal, but the patient complains of highly sensitive and spontaneously painful teeth).

Severe Grinding. As long as the jaw stays in dynamic movement (that is, the temporalis doesn't contract intensely enough to prevent any excursive or lateral movement of the mandible, but still provides significant resistance to lateral pterygoid activity), the lateral pterygoids can grind the teeth vigorously. Severe grinding results in obviously worn teeth, a stiff and sore jaw, sensitive teeth, and muscle pain when chewing.

Mild Grinding. When the temporalis muscle provides resistance (that is, mildly contracted, closing the teeth together), minimal effort is necessary for the lateral pterygoids to grind the teeth. Durations of these muscle contractions can be prolonged because neither the temporalis nor the lateral pterygoid muscles become tired. Over years teeth wear, but the person has no pain symptoms.

What's The Point?

So what's the point? One can have completely normal teeth and jaws with no tooth wear and still, complain of severe orofacial pain symptoms (the primary clencher). Further, another person may have severely worn teeth and no pain at all (the mild grinder). Ultimately, with bruxism, it doesn't matter how one's teeth or jaws are aligned. What matters is how intensely and frequently one clenches his or her teeth.

Treatment

Because bruxism is a condition of the muscles which move the jaw, dentistry has been charged with the responsibility of treating, and more importantly, preventing it.

Dentistry can be defined as the art and science of keeping teeth healthy, and the study of how they fit together. Consider a tooth with a substantial amount of decay. The dentist removes the diseased portion of the tooth (thereby prolonging its health) and then repairs the cavity with a restorative material. But the dentist isn't through yet. He then determines how the newly restored tooth fits against the opposing tooth in the opposite jaw when the mouth closes and during chewing. He confirms the two opposing teeth are compatible, or in other words, they don't traumatically occlude or touch, but work efficiently together during chewing. Anyone who's had a filling or crown knows what it's like for the tooth to hit "high" or strike too hard. The dentist has to adjust the occlusion until the restored tooth feels comfortable when the teeth bite together.

To treat bruxism, dentists prescribe a splint or dental mouthguard. Sometimes called a nightguard, these devices are designed to protect the teeth from the continual wear of grinding. Nightguards are especially helpful for the mild to severe grinder.

However, for the primary clencher, treatment is quite complex. Having little or no signs of tooth wear, but suffering with headaches, rarely are patients or dentists aware that they're a victim of primary clenching . . . night after night. To complicate matters further, these patients aren't suffering from malocclusion (or, a poor bite). Instead, primary clenchers suffer from clenching teeth together intensely, producing temporalis muscle fatigue and subsequently, headache pain.

Where the typical nightguard helps the grinder, *the same device often causes the primary clencher to **increase the intensity of his or her temporalis contraction.*** Splint therapy most often fails for the primary clencher and he either gives up and takes massive doses of over-the-counter medication or travels from doctor to doctor in search of relief from headaches.

Treatment for the excursive clencher lies somewhere in-between the grinder and primary clencher. If the lateral pterygoid muscles are active, moving the jaw side to side, then splint therapy has a fairly good chance to work. However, if the temporalis muscles contract the most, then splint therapy alone is inadequate. Then, we usually need additional treatment like medicine, biofeedback, counseling, physical therapy, chiropractic, or trigger point injections.

Additional Help for Clenching

There's a new treatment specifically designed to suppress clenching. Remember our definition of bruxism? Intense jaw-clenching (during sleep), with or without forcible lateral jaw movements, where the intensity of clenching dictates the severity of grinding. Therefore, it would seem logical that to treat and prevent bruxism we have to suppress clenching intensity.

A simple way of suppressing or decreasing clenching intensity is to use the jaw-opening reflex (JOR), also termed the myotactic reflex. The JOR is a muscular reflex which halts the closure of the jaw when the teeth come into contact with a solid object. Ever bite on a piece of bone in a hamburger? It's the JOR that tells you the bone in the meat shouldn't be there and if you continue to close, you'll break your tooth. Although your teeth are much harder than the piece of bone, the jaw-opening reflex, through a complex neurological reflex, forces you to stop biting and open your mouth quickly and unconsciously.

We're created with the same reflex if we bite our tongue while chewing. You know how much that hurts! If you bite your tongue, you immediately stop biting and quickly open your mouth.

With that in mind, it's no wonder that a primary clencher will continue to clench on their nightguard...it's simply because they can!

Research at UCLA has shown that those who are primary clenchers actually clench harder with the nightguard than without!

So how do we use the JOR to suppress clenching? Normal nightguards cover all the teeth of one dental arch. Research at UCLA has shown that those who are primary clenchers actually clench harder with the nightguard than without!

But by building an appliance to stimulate the JOR, we can actually suppress and in many cases, stop intense clenching. In July of 1998, the Food and Drug Administration (FDA) in the United States approved a product available to dentists with the following claim: "Prevents TMJ syndrome due to high pressure clenching . . ." Called the NTI Clenching Suppression System (NTI stands for Nociceptive Trigeminal Inhibition . . . a fancy name for the JOR), this device stimulates the jaw-opening reflex and prevents one from clenching intensely or for any length of time (Figure 11.2). If a primary clencher can't clench, then his or hers temporalis muscles won't become fatigued and guess what? No headache pain!

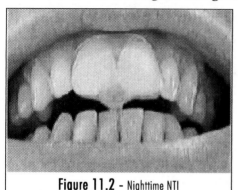

Figure 11.2 - Nighttime NTI

Teeth no longer are sensitive to cold temperatures. Best yet, we've discovered that *many migraine headache sufferers no longer have migraine headaches.*

That's right. We still don't know the exact cause (or, causes) of migraine headaches. However, current scientific research shows us there may be a direct connection between chronic, severely tensed temporalis muscles and if this condition can be arrested, migraines don't begin. And if migraines do start, using the NTI device significantly reduces the severity and frequency of these devastating headaches.

In June of 2001, the FDA accepted the NTI as an effective device that can *prevent* or *reduce* the effects of migraine headaches. This is so revolutionary! Now, many migraine patients can be safely treated, without side effects, with the NTI instead of costly drugs or injections.

Is The NTI Safe?

When fabricated properly by a dentist and used under his or her supervision, the NTI appliance is very safe. The NTI appliance is fitted on the upper front teeth (usually) and only one point contacts the lower front teeth. This small contact, just like biting on a piece of bone in food, stimulates the jaw-opening reflex and prevents a clencher from clenching, preventing the temporalis muscles from developing pain, and as the theory goes, headaches don't develop.

Some dentists are concerned that teeth may move if only the front teeth are covered. Research results show that such an appliance has to be worn continually for several days before any teeth will move. When properly used, the NTI is worn only when sleeping and once in a while when the patient is awake. But as long as teeth contact periodically during the day, teeth will not move.

If you're interested in the NTI appliance, contact http://www.nti-tts.com to locate a dentist in your area who's been trained to provide this revolutionary, anti-clenching device.

True Story

My Mystery

Maybe I should call this *My Journey*. About seven years ago, after my amalgams were removed, I developed problems with cavitations (I thought). I developed the most intense neck, ear, shoulder and back pain. It was unbearable at times. Life was really hard, to say the least. The pain kept me down.

Two weeks before seeing Dr. Shankland, I said goodbye to my family, left home, and planned my suicide. I parked on the railroad tracks and waited for an oncoming train . . . but for some reason, just couldn't.

I came to see Dr. Shankland. He understood the causes of my pain right away: bruxism and not cavitations! He made me an NTI appliance for nighttime and another appliance to wear during the day. After only one night, I knew he was right. I got up the next morning feeling like a different person!

I thank God first, then I thank God for Dr. Shankland giving me my like back. For anyone suffering . . . hold on and have faith. This is help! May God bless and guide you.

Glenda P.
Jamesville, NC
October 2001

References

1. **Harness DM, Peltier B:** *Comparison of MMPI scores with self-report of sleep disturbances and bruxism in the facial pain population.* J Craniomand Pract 1992;10:70-74.

2. **Allen JD, Rivera-Morales WC, Zwemer JD:** *The occurrence of temporomandibular disorder symptoms in healthy young adults with and without evidence of bruxism.* J Craniomand Pract 1990;8:312- 318.

3. **Kreisberg MK:** *Headache as a symptom of craniomandibular disorders* I: pathophysiology. J Craniomand Pract 1986;4:134-142.

4. **Shankland WE:** *Differential diagnosis of headaches.* J Craniomand Pract 1986;4:46-53.

5. **Boyd JP.** *Splitting the Headache.* Detroit: The Headache Prevention Institute, 1989.

6. **Shankland WE:** *Migraine and tension-type headache reduction through pericranial muscular suppression:* a preliminary report. J Craniomand Pract 2001;19:269-278.

Dr. James Boyd invented the NTI appliance. He conducts research concerning the indications and effects of this revolutionary appliance. He's a visionary and my friend. He and his family live in Southern California. Visit Dr. Boyd's web sites at: http://www.drjimboyd.com and http://www.NTI-TSS.com

Twelve

Medications

Until recently, using medicine to treat orofacial pain was ineffective at best, justifying Voltaire's comments: " . . . doctors pour drugs, of which they know little, for diseases of which they know less, into patients—of whom they know nothing."

In the past, when spontaneous remissions of pain occurred (which, is common with orofacial pain syndromes), medical practitioners argued that their potions produced the welcome relief from pain.

Some of the early medicines used were hemlock, quinine, strychnine and arsenic in the 17th century, which were replaced by ferrous carbonate, gelseminum powder, galvanic (electrical) therapy, potassium bromide, and x-radiation in the 18th and 19th centuries.

In our 20th century, such medicaments as trichloroethylene, B vitamins, nicotinic acid, amyl nitrite, cortisone, hormones, intravenous salicylate and iodine, intravenous typhoid vaccine, various muscle relaxants, and ultraviolet light have all been used.

In 1962, Blom reported the effective treatment of trigeminal neuralgia by using Tegretal, an anticonvulsant medication. Since then, we've discovered many drugs, all of which have improved our ability to treat medically orofacial pain disorders.

In this chapter, we'll discuss traditional (called allopathic) medical therapies for orofacial pain. That generally means treating segments of the trigeminal nerve. In chapter 13, we'll discuss various alternative medical treatments.

Anticonvulsants

Today, we no longer bleed patients with leaches (although, believe it or not, some researchers are recommending that again!) or plunge hands into hot water to treat trigeminal pain. Fortunately, in recent years, pharmaceutical manufacturers have produced several fine medicines, which help reduce or eliminate orofacial pain symptoms . . . at times.

Some medicines are used for more than one purpose. For example, two or three aspirins will relieve a headache, but ½ to 1 tablet every other day of this common anti-inflammatory drug reduces blood clotting, possibly preventing heart attacks. In fact, researchers now report that if a person takes an aspirin during a heart attack, his or her chances for recovery are vastly improved.

The same phenomenon occurs when we use anticonvulsant medications to treat orofacial pain. Anticonvulsant medications reduce the intensity and frequency of motor nerve firing by interfering with channels or specific sites in motor nerve fibers or by changing the activity of specific neurotransmitters. Changing any of these normal nerve functions reduces electrical activity of the nerves, and the nerves don't discharge erratically, causing muscles to contract uncontrollably.

Some anticonvulsants produce the same effects in sensory nerves, reducing the transmission of pain sensations to the brain. Granted, some sufferers of orofacial pain gain only reduced pain relief, but believe me, pain sufferers welcome any relief.

Currently, six (6) anticonvulsant medications are used to treat orofacial pain in the United States. Four are routinely prescribed, one provides limited but promising results, and one is, at the time of this writing, still in the experimental stages.

Tegretal. Tegretal, the first effective medication used to treat trigeminal neuralgia, often provides pain relief quickly and adequately. We also use Tegretal to gauge the severity of pain by observing how a patient reacts to different doses of medication.

Short-term side effects (Table 12.1) include drowsiness, fatigue, dizziness, nausea, twitching of the eyes, and memory loss. These side effects usually pass once the body adapts to the medication, except for drowsiness, which seems to be the main complaint of patients.

There's one major physiological problem with Tegretal: bone marrow cell damage. Bone marrow cells (stem cells), which produce the various types of blood cells, are susceptible to damage from Tegretal. For that reason, we order a blood test before starting a patient on Tegretal, with additional blood tests every few months to monitor any changes in these stem cells.

Never abruptly stop taking Tegretal, or else hallucinations and seizures may begin. Obviously, bone marrow damage and hallucinations are severe side effects. If, however, I can both reduce a patient's orofacial pain and monitor his or her blood, making sure that the cells remain healthy, these potential side effects are well worth the possible risks.

Table 12.1: Anticonvulsant drugs used also for the treatment of chronic orofacial pain.			
Trade Name	Generic Name	Usual Daily Dosage (mg)*	Most Common Side Effects
Tegretal	Carbama zepine	600-1200	Drowsiness, blurred vision, dizziness, damage to blood forming cells
Dilantin	Phenytoin	300-400	Drowsiness, dizziness, double vision, difficulty walking
Klonopin	Clonazepam	0.5 - 1.5	Aggressiveness, agitation, increased salivation, decreased sex drive
Neurontin	Gabapentin	50-60	Drowsiness, dizziness, gastrointestinal upset
Lamictal	Lamotrigine	100-200	Severe skin rash, double and/or blurred vision, headache, dizziness
Trileptal	Oxcarba-zepine	300-1200	Drowsiness, blurred vision, dizziness
*Dosages vary greatly			

Dilantin. Dilantin is commonly used to control the effects of epilepsy. Fortunately, like Tegretal, Dilantin also helps reduce orofacial neurological pain for some patients. It's often used in combination with Tegretal.

The side effects (Table 12.1) of Dilantin are drowsiness, fatigue, and gingival (gum) over-growth. If you're prescribed Dilantin, keep your teeth and ginginvae as clean as possible, and see your dentist every six months. If the gum tissues begin to grow, you'll require oral surgery to correct the problem.

Klonopin. I've found Klonopin to be very effective for treating patients suffering with orofacial pain, as well as a disorder termed myoclonic dyskinesia (uncontrolled, rhythmic muscle movement). Klonopin is used alone or in combination with other medications.

Short-term side effects (Table 12.1) of Klonopin include drowsiness, difficulty in walking, aggressiveness, and an increase in saliva.

Neurontin. Neurontin is a new medication and one which has helped many of my patients. Neurontin doesn't injure the liver, unlike most drugs.

Chief side effects of Neurontin (Table 12.1) are dizziness, sleepiness, fatigue, and nausea. Most, if not all of these symptoms, subside within a few days.

Lamictal. Used as an additional medication for epilepsy, Lamictal has recently been prescribed for trigeminal neuralgia, especially in combination with Tegretal. Although not used widely yet for orofacial pain, Lamictal is one more medication at our disposal to help these patients. Clinical studies show that Lamictal is effective in reducing the pain of diabetic neuropathy, phantom limb pain, and even the harsh disorder of sympathetically mediated pain (formerly known as sympathetic reflex dystrophy or RSD).

The main side effect of Lamictal is skin rash in about 10% of all those who take the medication. This rash has been fatal in a few cases, especially in pediatric patients.

Trileptal. Presently, Trileptal has recently been approved by the FDA for the treatment of pain. Similar to Tegretal in effect, it may hold great promise in the future to treat orofacial pain.

Antispasticity Medications

Currently, one antispasmotic drug on the market (in the US) works well in the treatment of orofacial pain. Baclofen resembles Tegretal and Dilantin because it reduces the excitation of nerve impulses in areas of the brain, which receive and process pain sensations. A late friend, Dr. Gerhard Fromm, was the chief clinical investigator for Baclofen and honored me by asking for my opinion of his scientific papers about Baclofen prior to their publication. So, I learned a lot about this medication while it was still in the experimental stages.

Lacking Tegretal's potential to harm the liver, Baclofen's chief side effects are drowsiness, dizziness, and gastrointestinal upset. If prescribed Baclofen, never stop taking it abruptly as hallucinations or seizures may occur.

Antidepressants

Antidepressants are another example of using a group of medications differently than how they were originally intended. These medications not only provide a sedative quality, but also inhibit the reabsorption or uptake of a major chemical in the pain puzzle serotonin. This chemical seems to play a very big role in the perception and perpetuation of pain.

The actual mechanism is complicated and far beyond the scope or intent of this book. Basically, serotonin is produced in specific areas in the brain. In the brain and spinal cord, serotonin dampens particular nerve fibers (the spinothalamic tract) from carrying pain sensations to the brain. These antidepressant drugs stop the removal of serotonin from nerve junctions, thus allowing for more pain suppression than normal. Therefore, these antidepressants are termed Selective Serotonin Reuptake Inhibitor (SSRI) drugs.

Most antidepressants are known as tricyclics due to their chemical structure. These drugs are used in pain management for several reasons, in addition to inhibiting serotonin removal. **First,** these medications are prescribed in such low doses that toxicity is not a concern.

Second, although they all produce similar side effects (namely, dry mouth, dizziness, and constipation), patients tolerate them well.

Third, because these antidepressant medications have a sedating effect, they're very useful with chronic pain patients because these poor sufferers generally also have insomnia.

Fourth and probably most important, since antidepressants don't produce the "high" or euphoria like many of the pain medications, abuse is not a problem.

The more common antidepressants used to treat orofacial pain are listed below. There are many similarities but yet, important differences, which need to be considered before recommending any of them to our patients. As with most medications, avoid drinking alcohol while taking antidepressants.

Elavil. Elavil is the most widely used antidepressant in pain management. I usually prescribe a starting dose of 10 milligrams (mg) to 25 mg at bedtime. The first morning or two drowsiness may occur, but that side effect is overcome in just a few days.

The two most frustrating side effects of Elavil (Table 12.2) are dry mouth, which generally doesn't go away, and weight gain due to water retention. Stop taking Elavil, and the water weight is usually lost quickly.

Prozac. Prozac is the most widely prescribed drug today in the world. It's especially helpful in treating orofacial pain patients who are also suffering with depression. Unfortunately, many of our pain patients also suffer with depression, especially if there's been a long history of failed diagnoses.

Some of the major side effects of Prozac (Table 12.2) are dry mouth, fatigue, dizziness, and reduced sexual interest.

Desyrel. Another popular and successful antidepressant, which we use to treat orofacial pain, is Desyrel (Trazazone), whose effects may take up to four weeks to occur, so pain reduction may be slow but steady. Like the other antidepressants, Desyrel is good at inhibiting the reuptake or reabsorption of serotonin in the brain and at the spinal cord level, thereby decreasing the perception of pain.

A typical side effect of all antidepressants is dry mouth (Table 12.2). Desyrel is no exception, but fortunately, this irritating problem isn't as prominent as with Elavil or Prozac.

Other side effects of Desyrel are dizziness, confusion, bad taste, and blurred vision. Men must avoid Desyrel as it may produce priapism (a condition of a prolonged and at times, permanent, painful erection).

Table 12.2: Common antidepressants used in the treatment of facial pain.			
Trade Name	Generic Name	Usual Daily Dosage(mg)*	Common Side Effects
Elavil	Amitriptyline	10-25 at bed	Dry mouth, drowsiness, fatigue, water retention
Prozac	Fluoxetine	10-20	Dry mouth, fatigue, dizziness, decreased sex drive
Desyrel	Trazodone	50-100	Dizziness, confusion, bad taste, blurred vision
Pamelor	Nortriptyline	25-75	Dry mouth, constipation, increase in appetite, bad taste
Tofranil	Imipramine	75-150	Dry mouth, bad taste, increase in appetite, fatigue
*For pain relief only; not for depression			

Pamelor. Unlike the other tricyclic antidepressants, Pamelor (nortriptyline) is packaged as a capsule, which is the only type some people can swallow.

Possible side effects (Table 12.2), which usually go away during treatment, include dry mouth, constipation, an increase in appetite, especially for sweets and unpleasant taste. Like the others, don't discontinue the use of Pamelor abruptly and without first consulting your doctor. I prefer this medication for most of my patients who require an antidepressant.

Tofranil. Tofranil is an older but still reliable tricyclic antidepressant medication. Like Desyrel, it may take several weeks for the benefits of pain reduction to be noticed, and therefore, don't stop taking Tofranil abruptly.

Some of Tofranil's major side effects (Table 12.2) are dry mouth, unpleasant taste, and an increase in appetite especially for sweet foods.

NSAIDs

Most of you reading this chapter are most familiar with this classification of medications, the Non-Steroidal Anti-inflammatory Drugs. Aspirin and ibuprofen are the most common NSAIDs.

NSAIDs work both in the central nervous system to reduce fever and at the site of injury to reduce inflammation, pain and swelling.

After any type of tissue injury, a complex set of chemical reactions changes acrachidonic acid into a classification of irritants called prostaglandins, which stimulate pain receptors and produce pain.

NSAIDs apparently interrupt this cascade of chemical reactions by inhibiting the action of a very important enzyme, cyclooxygenase (termed COX-1 enzyme), which prevents the formation of prostaglandins. That's why it's important to take aspirin or ibuprofen at regular intervals (usually, every 6 hours), in order to keep the level of the NSAIDs at an effective, consistent level.

Obviously, the problems of gastrointestinal injury, stomach upset, and decreased blot clotting are common side effects of taking NSAIDs for any length of time. These problems are often magnified because chronic pain patients have either taken medications for years or, due to chronic anxiety, chronic pain patients frequently have gastric problems. I face this problem of giving medication daily. Doctors walk a fine line between the therapeutic benefits of the drugs we prescribe and their potential of dangerous side effects.

A pharmacological revolution is now occurring in pain medications. The Food and Drug Administration (FDA) recently approved a new classification of drugs, COX-2 enzyme inhibitors. Remember the chemical breakdown of arachidonic acid mentioned above? An enzyme (cyclooxygenase or COX-1) was key in this reaction. We now know that a second enzyme, COX-2 or cyclooxygenase 2, may be the real enzyme responsible for producing the protaglandins that cause pain.

Research shows separate mechanisms produce two different forms of cyclooxygenase enzymes. COX-1 is stimulated by normal body physiology, its concentration remains constant, and COX-1 is present in most tissues. The normal process of inflammation begins with arachidonic acid, an unsaturated fatty acid obtained from animal fats in our diets. This acid is converted by COX-1 to prostaglandins, which stimulate many other regulatory functions (e.g., stomach mucous production and cellular division, kidney sodium excretion and renal blood flow, platelet formation) and generalized inflammation production. NSAIDs suppress COX-1 ability to synthesize prostaglandins, thereby inhibiting essential body functions as well as the production of inflammation.

The exciting news is this: New drugs which target the COX-2 enzyme inhibit only inflammatory prostaglandin formation, thereby avoiding the potential dangerous side effects of today's NSAIDs.

It appears that, unlike the COX-1 enzyme, COX-2 is induced by the action of macrophages, the scavenger white blood cells, which arrive very quickly after tissue injury. A drug selective to stop the activity of the COX-2 enzyme would be safer, and higher doses could theoretically be given to improve pain suppression and stop inflammation.

I know that these tidbits of biochemistry are a little complicated. To summarize:

- The COX-1 enzyme continually produces various prostaglandins used for many essential bodily functions, the production of inflammation and pain being only two

- The COX-2 enzyme is induced by macrophages after tissue injury to produce specific prostaglandins, which cause inflammation and subsequent pain

- Regular NSAIDs inhibit the action of COX-1, therefore reducing inflammation production, but also injuring other normal cellular functions

- The new NSAIDs appear to block the action of COX-2, which is specific for inflammation only, making these medications much safer

Today, two COX-2 inhibitor drugs have been approved by the FDA: Celebrex (Searle Pharmaceuticals) and Vioxx (Merck Co.). At least 20.7 million Americans suffer from osteoarthritis, for which these drugs are initially recommended because the sufferers have to take NSAIDs for their entire life times. Our patients with orofacial pain greatly benefit also, from these and other COX-2 medications, most of which are still being developed.

Just recently, the FDA has approved the use of COX-2 inhibitor drugs for the treatment of acute pain. That's great because I've had tremendous success using these new COX-2 inhibitors in the treatment of pain especially caused by various types of arthritis, but also in treating joint inflammation.

A word of caution. While writing this chapter, news was released about possible serious side effects of COX-2 inhibitor drugs: They may increase the risk of heart attack, stroke, and blood clotting disorders. In a study presented to the National Academy of Science in January, 1999, researchers reported that COX-2 inhibitors, at least in mice, suppressed a hormone-like substance, prostacyclin. This substance is required to dilate blood vessels and inhibit clotting. It was suggested that many older patients who may take COX-2 inhibitors for arthritis may see an increase in heart attack, stroke, and blood clotting disorders. This is only a preliminary report and found, at the time of this writing, only in genetically engineered mice to be unable to use prostacyclin properly. In human beings, these side effects may never be a problem.

Let's discuss the major NSAIDs (COX-1 inhibitors . . . you now know what that is, don't you?). Remember that many of the newer COX-2 inhibitors may not be publicly available for a few years yet, so we still need to use the NSAIDs available to us today.

Before proceeding, realize that most of the NSAIDs, when taken for any length of time, have the potential to cause tinnitus, or ringing in the ears. Many patients with orofacial pain and temporomandibular joint problems also experience tinnitus as one symptom, causing the sufferer to see many doctors when discontinuing the use of the NSAID will stop the ringing in the ears.

Aspirin. Believe it or not, aspirin is still the medication of choice to treat mild to moderate pain, inflammation, and fever (for adults). Like all NSAIDs, aspirin works by inhibiting the cyclooxygenase-1 (COX-1) enzyme in the production of certain prostaglandin chemicals, which ultimately produce inflammation and subsequent pain.

Aspirin is a trade name for acetylsalicylic acid, a common analgesic. The Greek physician Hippocrates in the fifth century B.C. used a form of the drug: powder extracted from the bark of willows to treat pain and reduce fever.

Salicin, the parent of the salicylate drug family, was successfully isolated in 1829 from willow bark. Sodium salicylate, a predecessor to aspirin, was developed along with salicylic acid in 1875 as a pain reliever. However, sodium salicylate irritated the lining of the stomach, so its use was limited. In 1897, Felix Hoffman, a German chemist, who was working for the Bayer Chemical Company, had been using the sodium salicylate to treat his father's arthritis. The sodium salicylate caused his father severe stomach pain, so Hoffman prepared a less acidic chemical. This new buffered aspirin was acetylsalicylic acid. Today we know this very same aspirin preparation as Bayer Aspirin.

Are Bayer or Bufferin aspirin the best on the market? Not at all! Aspirin is aspirin. Period. Many aspirins use buffering to reduce injury to the stomach lining. Caffeine is added to improve the activity of the chemical, acetylsalicylic acid.

If you have stomach problems, take coated aspirin, which will dissolve in your intestines, sparing your stomach lining further injury.

If you're prescribed a pain medication, you can improve the drug's effect by taking a couple of aspirin with the medication, thus improving the desired effects of pain reduction without increasing the side effects of the prescription drug. But first, check with your doctor before doing so for many reasons.

Aspirin comes as close to being a wonder drug as any medication on the market, yet it does cause side effects, primarily gastrointestinal irritation (nausea, heartburn, stomach bleeding and pain). It's been implicated in Reye syndrome, a rare but occasionally fatal condition in children or teenagers suffering with chickenpox or the flu. Aspirin has also been associated with hemorrhagic (bleeding) stroke in a small percentage of patients who use the drug regularly, although the majority of regular users have no problem with any type of internal bleeding.

Aspirin should be used cautiously with patients suffering with uncontrolled high blood pressure, liver or kidney disease, peptic ulcer, or other conditions, which might increase the risk of cerebral hemorrhage or other internal bleeding.

A Personal note. In April 1999, I was honored to speak to several of Bayer's scientists at their home office and plant located outside of Colgne, Germany. What a sense of history, being in the very facility where Bayer aspirin was first formulated: Dr. Jim Boyd and I spoke concerning the theoretical basis for using the NTI appliance (Chapter 11).

Ibuprofen. An NSAID, advertised as less injurious to your stomach lining is ibuprofen, sold under various trade names (Motrin, Motrin IB, Nuprin, and Advil, just to name the more popular products). Like all NSAIDs, ibuprofen works by inhibiting the COX-1 enzyme, thus limiting the production of certain prostaglandins. Again, the interruption of the COX-1 enzyme appears to ultimately result in the reduction of fever, inflammation and swelling, and pain perception.

Although you can purchase ibuprofen as an OTC (over-the-counter) drug, you need to take a prescription dosage of 2400 to 3200 mg per day in divided doses. If you take it for any length of time, check with your doctor.

Ibuprofen has gained much popularity because its manufacturers claim ibuprofen is safer to the stomach lining than aspirin. True, but exactly how much safer? Although ibuprofen reduces irritation to the stomach lining and thereby lessens stomach bleeding, these unfortunate side effects still occur with ibuprofen, but just slightly less than with aspirin.

Other side effects are vertigo, headaches, skin rashes, and an elevation of liver enzymes (damage to liver with chronic use) in the blood. Fortunately, dangerous kidney complications (water and salt retention, acute kidney failure), hepatitis, and general hypersensitive reactions (fever, hypertension, aseptic meningitis) are rare with ibuprofen.

Dangerous complications (bleeding ulcers, perforations) are not common with ibuprofen.

Naprosyn. Until recently, Naprosyn was a prescription medication (in the US). Now, sold as an OTC drug (e.g., Aleve), Naprosyn is an effective NSAID. You take this medication less often than aspirin or ibuprofen. In theory, this tends to keep the blood levels of the chemical more consistent.

As with the other OTC NSAIDs, you need to take prescription strength of Naprosyn in order to achieve a therapeutic (or effective) level in the blood. Generally sold as Anaprox and Anaprox DS, you need to take 275 mg to 550 mg three times per day.

Common side effects of Naprosyn are heartburn, constipation, abdominal pain, tinnitus, and hearing disturbances.

Also, like all NSAIDs, Naprosyn has the potential for causing kidney damage. I'm concerned about the amounts of these easily obtainable medications being consumed today. There will probably be a lot of work for transplant surgeons in the next few decades.

Naprelan. Naprelan, a prescription NSAID, is a similar formulation to Naprosyn or Anaprox, except Naprelan is time-released.

Daypro. Daypro is an effective NSAID, which is available as a prescription medication only. I like to prescribe Daypro because you take two tablets each morning and that's it. Daypro is primarily indicated for long-term use. You don't have to worry about when to take the next dose. I've also not had many patients complain about side effects such as stomach pain from Daypro.

As with most medications which need to be taken for prolonged periods, it's a good idea to have your doctor check your blood chemistry from time to time. In about 1% of those taking Daypro, liver injury has been reported.

Other side effects of Daypro are similar to NSAIDs: gastrointestinal upset, tinnitus, and kidney injury, which may be permanent.

Table 12.3: Non-Steroidal Anti-inflammatory Drugs (NSAIDs).				
Drug Type	Brand Names	Generic Names	Desired Effects	Side Effects
Aspirin	Aspirin, Bufferin, Ascripton, Ecotrin, Empirin, Anacin	Acetylsalicylic acid	Reduce: Pain, Inflammation, Fever, Swelling	Stomach Irritation; Prolonged bleeding; Tinnitus
Non-NSAID	Tylenol, Datril, Anacin II Ultram*	Acetamenophen Tramadol	Reduce: Pain, Fever	Liver damage; Kidney damage
NSAID	Motrin, Advil, Motrin IB Aleve	Ibuprofen Naproxen sodium	Reduce: Fever, Pain, Inflammation, Swelling	Stomach irritation; Dizziness; Prolonged bleeding; interference with calcium channel blocking drugs; Tinnitus
NSAID*	Anaprox, Naprosyn Naprelan, Daypro, Toradol, Lodine, Arthrotec, Anadaid, Cataflam Orudis Feldene Relafin	Naproxen sodium Naproxen sodium Oxaprozin Ketorolac acid Etodolac acid Diclofenac sodium Flurbriprofen Dicolfenac potssium Ketoprofen Piroxicam Nabumetone	Reduce: Fever, Pain, Inflammation, Swelling	Stomach irritation; Dizziness; Prolonged Bleeding; interference with calcium channel blocking drugs; Tinnitus
*Prescription medications				

Ultram. Ultram, a new and effective analgesic, was approved in 1995 by the FDA. It isn't an NSAID, but rather a prescription analgesic in a classification of its own. Ultram's an interesting drug and works two different ways. First, Ultram binds with and activates opiate receptors in the brain (making the brain act as if opium, a very strong narcotic, was present), thus producing pain relief. Second, Ultram also stops the reabsorption of both serotonin and norepinephrine, which both produce analgesia at the spinal cord level.

Ultram is an excellent pain medication, not only due to its fast and efficient activity, but also because, unlike narcotics, which produce similar pain relief, Ultram doesn't depress the respiration rate. This is very important because death by overdose is virtually impossible. Understand that working with chronic pain patients, we have to consider the possibility of suicide.

Our greatest concern with Ultram is the potential for addiction in those who are prone to addiction to alcohol, hypnotics, centrally acting analgesics, opioids or psychotropic drugs. In other words, we prescribe Ultram sparingly to patients who have had addiction problems or those who tend to exhibit addictive personalities.

Other side effects are dizziness, nausea, headache, constipation, and insomnia. Fortunately, most of my patients get over these side effects if they can stick with Ultram for a day or so. This medication may be used in combination with other prescribed pain-relief medications.

I've found that Ultram either works or it doesn't. There's no inbetween. You can greatly improve the action of Ultram by taking one or two acetaminophen tablets along with the Ultram.

Acetaminophen. Like Ultram, acetaminophen (i.e., Tylenol) is an analgesic not classified as an NSAID. Both Ultram and acetaminophen reduce pain, but neither reduces inflammation like the NSAIDs. Acetaminophen also helps lower elevated body temperatures. In fact, acetaminophen is just as effective as aspirin in both analgesia (pain reduction) and antipyretic (reducing fever) qualities.

I find acetaminophen, like Ultram, either works or it doesn't. My clinical experience shows me that some patients refuse to try acetaminophen because they wrongly think that it's inferior to aspirin or ibuprofen. Not true.

Acetaminophen is an excellent analgesic for those with stomach problems and those allergic to either aspirin or ibuprofen. Like aspirin, acetaminophen can be combined with narcotic medications to form potent pain-killing drugs. Also, for children and young adults, acetaminophen is the drug of choice instead of aspirin or ibuprofen.

My main concern about acetaminophen is that, since it's not a prescription medication, most people unknowingly think the side effects are harmless. This couldn't be further from the truth. Taking acetaminophen for prolonged periods may produce liver damage and actual liver death. In addition, kidneys are also damaged by acetaminophen taken for long periods of time. Remember this, if you must take acetaminophen for any length of time, talk with your doctor about these potential, serious side effects.

Narcotics

Narcotics are termed opiate agonists. In the brain, narcotics combine with opiate receptors which produce pain suppression. Opiate drugs are named after their natural source, the opium poppy which contains several active chemicals such as morphine and codeine. Examples of synthetic opiates are meperidine (Demerol) and methadone. Both natural and synthetic narcotics are classified by the Drug Enforcement Agency (DEA) according to their potential for abuse.

For example, heroin is classified as a Schedule I drug because of its high potential for abuse. These drugs bind to opiate receptors throughout the central nervous system which causes the release of endorphins and enkephlins, the body's natural opiates to reduce or suppress pain perception. Schedule I drugs are available only for research purposes. Most of the narcotics we prescribe are classified as Schedule II (e.g., plain codeine or Demerol), Schedule III (e.g., acetaminophen with codeine), or Schedule IV (e.g., Darvocet).

Narcotics, the most effective prescription medicines we have today to control pain, are frequently combined with aspirin, acetaminophen, and recently, with ibuprofen, improving the potency without increasing the amount of the narcotic. Empirin (aspirin added) Compound with Codeine, Tylenol with Codeine, and Vicoprofen (ibuprofen added) are examples. Darvocet is another example, with the combination of Darvon and acetaminophen.

Aside from the addictive potentials, the major complication with narcotics is depression of respiration. These drugs can slow or even stop breathing if taken in large quantities. This is especially true if alcohol is consumed with a narcotic. That's why Ultram pleases me: Its ability to reduce pain is equal to many narcotics without depressing the respiration.

Also, narcotics produce constipation, drowsiness, and stomach problems. Ideally, we like to prescribe narcotics for acute, not chronic pain conditions, or as a rescue medicine for severe episodes of pain.

Cortisone

Cortisone is an anti-inflammatory medication prescribed to reduce inflammation quickly. Unfortunately, cortisone has many side effects and should be used sparingly. Weight gain, liver and kidney damage are just a few reasons why I limit my use of cortisone. Far too many prescriptions are written primarily because cortisone makes one feel so good so quickly.

We're also very concerned about the activity of cortisone in the development of NICO lesions of the jaws (see Chapter 7). These dead areas of bone may be linked to chronic cortisone use. We're still researching this, but for this reason alone, I try to avoid prescribing cortisone whenever I can.

Many of us substitute a natural anti-inflammatory medication, Sarapin, for cortisone. Sarapin exhibits all the good, anti-inflammatory properties as cortisone without the adverse reactions.

Local Anesthetics

If asked about local anesthetics, immediately you'd think of Novocaine that your dentist uses to numb areas of your mouth. That's only partially correct. Novocaine (procaine) is basically used only for injecting skeletal muscle trigger points today. More effective and safer local anesthetics have been created since Novocaine's birth in 1905.

We use local anesthetics primarily to diagnose, not treat orofacial pain. Just because an area hurts doesn't mean that the problem is located there. If your doctor doesn't derive a proper diagnosis, you may undergo an unnecessary or improper surgical procedure. Local anesthetic injections are probably the most important testing procedure that I perform several times a day.

Just like turning off the specific circuit breaker or fuse, local anesthetic injections are used to numb various structures in an attempt to discover what, if any, structure or structures might be causing pain.

We also use local anesthetic injections to treat skeletal muscle trigger points, or small, chronic muscle spasms.

If you remember nothing else from this book, please burn this into your mind: if you're in pain, don't allow anyone to operate or perform any invasive procedure without first turning the pain off with a local anesthetic injection. Demand it if the doctor recommends a root canal or surgery or tooth removal. It's your body and you have a right to obtain a proper diagnosis, and then your treatment options must be explained to you. If your doctor refuses to demonstrate by local anesthetic where your pain originates, get out of that office, and find a doctor who will work with and for you.

I can't emphasize this point strongly enough. It's a tragedy so many patients end up in my office who never, ever had an anesthetic injection before undergoing surgery. I'm ashamed of my profession for this irresponsible approach to patient care.

Muscle Relaxants

Another very important group of medications that we use in treating orofacial pain is muscle relaxants. These drugs are used to relax skeletal muscles primarily of the head and neck.

Table 12.4: Common skeletal muscle relaxants.				
Brand Name	**Generic Name**	**Usual Daily Dosage**	**Desired Effects**	**Side Effects**
Skelaxin	Metaxalone	1-2 every 6 hrs	Relax muscles; reduce pain	Stomach upset; Drowsiness
Parafon Forte DSC	Chlorzoxazone	1-2 every 6 hrs	Same as above	Same as above
Flexeril	Cyclobenzaprine	1 every 8 hrs	Same as above	Same as above
Soma	Carisoprodol	1 every 6 hrs	Same as above	Same as above

Many doctors and patients alike shy away from using muscle relaxants because of the general sedative effects many, by not all, produce. Since the late 1950s, when Soma was introduced, muscle relaxants have been very helpful, but since they produced such strong sedation, they had to be cautiously (or, should have been!) prescribed. In 1977, Flexeril was released for public use, and it was an improvement. However, even Flexeril causes sedation, and I only prescribe this muscle relaxant when I purposely want to sedate a patient.

Although the FDA approved it in 1962, only in the last few years has Skelaxin been reintroduced. As with Ultram, I've been very excited about Skelaxin because it's so effective in relieving muscle pain, and it rarely produces any sedation.

I'm a prime example of my own doctoring. I'm very susceptible to most medications. If I take any OTC allergy drugs (e.g., Benadryl or Pseudophed), I'm asleep within 45 minutes. As I can't afford to be sedated, I can take two Skelaxin tablets every 4 to 6 hours and only feel better with no sedation. Understand that people are variable, but I rarely find patients who don't also have success with Skelaxin. If you're prescribed another muscle relaxant, you might want to suggest Skelaxin to your doctor.

Another excellent, non-sedating muscle relaxant that I often prescribe is Parafon forte DSC. Like Skelaxin, Parafon forte provides excellent pain relief without sedation.

Chapter Summary

All medications produce side effects; few are good. As doctors, we understand and utilize that fact. As our research improves, our drugs also improve with fewer side effects.

As a consumer, you must be aware of the potential side effects of any drugs prescribed for you. Be honest (and fair) with your doctor(s) concerning medications that you're currently taking when a new one is prescribed. Don't forget to tell the doctor about supplements and vitamins that you're also taking, because some prescription medications don't mix well with certain supplements.

Follow the directions for any prescription drug and report immediately any unusual side effects. Trust me, the doctor wants to be bothered with this information, as it may be life threatening to you.

CHAPTER Thirteen

Alternative Treatment

Today, western medicine is experiencing a revolution. Battle lines, drawn between traditional or allopathic medicine and non-traditional or naturopathic (alternative) medicine, are slowly being erased. Traditionally trained dentists, physicians and podiatrists are criticized by many who promote and practice the various types of alternative therapies for not being more progressive and less traditional. It's interesting that a recent national magazine conducted a survey, the results of which were startling: Over 55% of us seek alternative health care before consulting a traditional doctor. Medical views have to change. In 1992, Congress ordered the National Institute of Health, the premier biological-research organization on earth, to establish the Office of Alternative Medicine.

If alternative medicine is gaining so much in popularity then an honest question is, "If alternative medicine is so effective, why don't allopathic doctors embrace it?" There are several honest answers to this probing question.

First, doctors practice as they were taught, and most medical and dental professors teach as they were taught. That's just the way it is. For example, one of our courses in physiological chemistry was entitled "Nutrition." After the professor gave his introduction to his first lecture, he announced, "That, ladies and gentlemen, is the extent of education our medical students receive concerning nutrition." Imagine that? About 10 minutes and that's all! Western medicine has forgotten the value

Doctors practice as they were taught and most medical and dental professors teach as they were taught.

of proper nutrition and now relies upon the wonders of modern chemistry and pharmacology.

Second, as students, we were taught that one receives all the vitamins and minerals needed in a normal diet. Does that even make sense? Think of all the fast and processed foods we consume today. Nutrients are lost. Proteins are denatured (structurally destroyed), and vitamin therapy is considered a joke by the traditional health care system. In fact, those of us who recommend vitamin therapy are often ridiculed and called quacks by medical educators and state boards of dentistry and medicine.

Third, traditional medicine and dentistry have divided the body into groups of specialties and rarely view the human body as whole, a total organism. We're forced to view our particular portion of the body only, and most of us rarely consider other organ systems, especially on the cellular level. We treat symptoms and not causes. Preventing diseases is not a consideration because that's the way we were taught.

Fourth, the standard of care in Western medicine doesn't include alternative therapies . . . yet. Malpractice is a real fear among doctors. If we treat a patient with alternative therapy and he or she doesn't respond, our colleagues are very quick to criticize our choice of therapy and even encourage the patient to seek legal advice or, at the very least, turn us into our respective state boards. These colleagues quickly forget that traditional therapies also often fail, but that's considered standard of care and not quackery.

It's time to consider both traditional and alternative therapies as we seek to help our patients with their health care. After all, it's the patient's choice, not ours.

Naturopathy

Naturopathic medicine, sometimes called naturopathy, is one of the oldest forms of healing. In the United States, the naturopathic medical profession's infrastructure is based on accredited educational institutions, professional licensing by a growing number of states, national standards of practice and care, peer review, and scientific research. Naturopathic physicians (NDs) receive extensive training in and use therapies that are primarily natural, hence, the name naturopathic. NDs also use clinical nutrition, homeopathy, botanical medicine, hydrotherapy, physical medicine, and counseling. Many NDs have additional training and certification in acupuncture and home birthing. The word naturopathy was first used in the US about 100 years ago, but the natural therapies and the philosophy on which naturopathy is based have been effectively used to treat diseases since ancient times.

The earliest doctors and healers worked with herbs, foods, water, fasting, and tissue manipulation -- gentle treatments that don't inhibit the body's own healing powers. Today's naturopathic physicians continue to use these therapies as their main tools and to advocate a healthy dose of primary prevention. In addition, modern NDs conduct and make practical use of the latest biochemical research involving nutrition, botanicals, homeopathy, and other natural treatments.

Naturopathic medicine was popular and widely available throughout the US well into the early part of the 20th century. Around 1920 there were a number of naturopathic medical schools and thousands of naturopathic physicians. But the rise of scientific medicine, the discovery and increasing use of drugs like antibiotics, the institutionalization of a large medical system all contributed to the temporary decline of naturopathic medicine and most other methods of natural healing.

However, by the 1970s, the American public was becoming increasingly disenchanted with conventional medicine. The profound clinical limitations of conventional medicine and its out-of-control costs were becoming obvious, and millions of Americans were inspired to look for "new" options and alternatives. Naturopathy and all of complementary alternative medicine began to enter a new era of rejuvenation. Today, licensed naturopathic physicians are experiencing noteworthy clinical successes, providing leadership in innovative natural medical research, and enjoying increasing political influence. In 1992, the National Institute of Health's (NIH) Office of Alternative Medicine, created by an act of Congress, invited leading naturopathic physicians (educators, researchers, and clinical practitioners) to serve on key federal advisory panels and to help define priorities and design protocols for state-of-the-art alternative medical research. The number of new NDs is steadily increasing, and licensure of naturopathic physicians is expanding into new states. By April of 1996, eleven of fifty states had naturopathic licensing laws (Alaska, Arizona, Connecticut, Hawaii, Maine, Montana, New Hampshire, Oregon, Utah, Vermont, and Washington). A number of other states are likely to enact naturopathic licensing in the near future.

The current scope of naturopathic practice includes:

- **Clinical Nutrition.** Many medical conditions can be treated more effectively with foods and nutritional supplements than they can by other means, with fewer complications and side effects. Naturopathic physicians use dietetics, natural hygiene, fasting, and nutritional supplementation in practice.

- **Botanical Medicine.** Many plant substances are powerful medicines. Where single chemically-derived drugs may only address a single problem, botanical medicines are able to address a variety of problems simultaneously. Their organic nature makes botanicals compatible with the body's own chemistry; hence, they can be gently effective with few toxic side effects.

- **Homeopathic Medicine.** Homeopathic medicine is based on the principle of like cures like (see below). It works on a subtle yet powerful electromagnetic level, gently acting to strengthen the body's healing and immune response.

- **Physical Medicine.** Naturopathic medicine has its own methods of therapeutic manipulation of muscles, bones, and spine. NDs also use ultrasound, diathermy, exercise, massage, water, heat and cold, air, and gentle electrical pulses.

- **Oriental Medicine.** According to the American Naturopathic Medical Association, oriental medicine is a complimentary healing philosophy to naturopathic medicine.

- **Naturopathic Obstetrics.** Naturopathic physicians provide natural childbirth care in an out-of-hospital setting. They offer prenatal and postnatal care using modern diagnostic techniques.

- **Psychological Medicine.** Mental attitudes and emotional states may influence, or even cause, physical illness. Naturopaths use counseling, nutritional balancing, stress management, hypnotherapy, biofeedback, and other therapies to help patients heal on the psychological level.

- **Minor Surgery.** As general practitioners, NDs perform in-office minor surgery, including repair of superficial wounds, removal of foreign bodies, cysts, and other superficial masses.

Homeopathy

Homeopathy was founded in the late nineteenth century by the German physician Samuel Hahnemann. Experienced in pharmacology, public health and industrial toxicology, Dr. Hahnemann was repulsed by such barbaric practices of the times as blood letting (using leaches to suck blood from sick patients) and applying mercury as an antiseptic. He dedicated himself to find effective, safer ways to treat patients.

Dr. Hahnemann experimented by chewing cinchona, a Peruvian bark known in the 19th century as a cure for malaria. He soon noticed that after chewing cinchona, he developed periodic fevers, similar to those characteristic of malaria. When he stopped chewing the bark, his fevers ceased. He theorized that if large doses caused malaria-like symptoms, then a small doses might stimulate the body to fight a specific disease. He experimented for years with many different substances and found similar results.

Based upon his years of research, Dr. Hahnemann developed the basic principles of homeopathy, which are as follows:

- Law of Similars (like cures like)

- Law of the Infinitesimal Dose (the more a substance is diluted, the greater its potency)

- An illness is specific to the individual

All these principles smack in the face of reason . . . for we doctors trained in traditional medicine. We're taught in pharmacology that generally, the higher the dose, the greater the effectiveness of the drug. But homeopathy purports the opposite: The more a substance is diluted, the greater its strength (or, higher its potency). Homeopathy also believes that the epidemic nature of chronic diseases we experience today is a direct result of the suppression of symptoms of diseases through modern, allopathic medical techniques.

How could this be true? The answer may be the electromagnetic frequency of the original molecules. Some researchers in quantum physics believe that if the original disease's electromagnetic frequency is matched (the Law of Similars), the body's defense mechanisms are stimulated to natural healing, without the toxic effects of medications.

In defense of homeopathy, there are currently a lot of research efforts aimed at identifying the frequencies of all types of substances, both living tissues and bacteria, in an attempt to match the specific frequencies for therapeutic purposes. If these researchers are successful, they'll ultimately prove scientifically the validity of homeopathy.

Do you have to see a doctor to benefit from homeopathic remedies? While it's always good to consult your doctor before using any medication, you can also get good information from many employees of health food stores. There, you'll see individual homeopathic remedies as well as formulations of more than one remedy. The packages will explain the condition the remedy treats, but you should consult your physician, especially one trained in homeopathy. The symbol x indicates the number of times the remedy has been diluted. Remember, one of the tenants of homeopathy is the Law of the Infinitesimal Dose (the more a substance is diluted, the greater its potency). Therefore, a 6x preparation means the solution has been diluted 6 times.

Some of the common remedies for pain are:

- **Arnica Montana 6x.** This is one of the most commonly recommended homeopathic pain remedies (especially for acute pain), the resorption of blood in cases of trauma and promotion of good circulation. It's contained in the formulation of Traumeel

- **Aconitum Napellus 12x.** Most effective when used immediately after an injury, Aconitum 12x reduces severe pain, like that of burns and surgery. It's also beneficial for arthritis and neuralgia

- **Chamonilla 3x.** A derivative of the calming herb chamomile, this remedy is good for the treatment of low-level chronic pain

- **Apis Mellifica 12x.** Good for treating inflammation, use this for insect bites, too

- **Hypercium Perforatum 6x.** Good for cuts and scrapes and head pain

- **Rhus Toxicodendron 6x.** Excellent for muscle pain, many sufferers of orofacial, ear and fibromyalgia pain can benefit from this remedy

- **Causticum.** Good for head pain and muscle tension

It's best to consult a homeopath before using these remedies because you might need to dilute the remedy's staring strength.

Chiropractic

I hesitate to consider chiropractic treatment as a type of alternative medicine. Of all alternative modes of therapy, I recommend chiropractic the most. In fact, I don't know how I could practice without my network of chiropractic physicians. Chiropractors are dedicated to aligning the body to stimulate its natural, inherent ability to heal itself.

Spinal adjustment has been practiced for centuries. In 1895, Daniel Palmer, a student of human anatomy and physiology, founded the profession of chiropractic. Apparently,

Palmer found a misaligned vertebra in a man's cervical (neck) spine. The man had been deaf for 17 years following a neck injury. Palmer performed what's termed a thrusting maneuver in that area of the neck and the man's hearing was restored.

Since that time, the professions of chiropractic and allopathic medicine have been at war. Traditionally, doctors of medicine were taught that chiropractors were nothing but quacks. Chiropractic doctors were taught that medical doctors over-treated with drugs and surgery, interrupting the body's innate intelligence, or the thought that all vital functions flow through the central nervous system. By treating spinal bony segments which impinged spinal nerves, the cause of an interrupted nervous flow would be treated and not just the symptoms.

Many chiropractors also use homeopathy and nutritional therapy to treat various types of disorders which may or may not be related to misalignment of the spinal column.

Chiropractic treatment is gaining respect from the medical profession and great acceptance from the general public. In a two-year study conducted by the British Medical Research Council, chiropractic treatment was found to be more successful than hospital out-patient treatment for low back pain.

Another study's results revealed that chiropractic treatment is effective for the treatment of headache pain, especially tension-type headaches. Further, chiropractic treatment is effective in treating carpal-tunnel syndrome, premenstrual syndrome, and temporomandibular joint problems. Virtually any joint or musculoskeletal problem, which will respond to conservative therapy, can be treated effectively by a chiropractor.

Many cervical nerve disorders (e.g., lesser and greater occipital nerve neuralgia) produce facial, eye and headache pain. If you experience pain in these areas, consult a chiropractor, especially before you consider any type of surgery.

A Personal note. My father is a medical doctor, so I was raised with the attitude that chiropractors were quacks, unworthy to be called Doctor. My wife's family, on the other hand, visited their family chiropractor often. While working one evening, I lifted a heavy box and injured by back. I could hardly walk the next day. My wife drug me kicking and screaming to a chiropractic physician. I was terrified, knowing that I'd probably be paralyzed if the doctor touched my back!

Was I ever surprised! Not only did I receive the finest physical examination I'd ever had, but the doctor immediately found the subluxation (a vertebra out of place, squeezing a spinal nerve) and adjusted my lower back painlessly. Immediately, my pain was gone, and I've been a believer in chiropractors ever since. By the way, my dad is now a believer, too!

Today, I couldn't practice without the help of a chiropractor for my TMJ and orofacial pain patients. Not only do my patients improve quicker with chiropractic

> *I don't know how I could practice without my network of chiropractic physicians.*

treatment, but their overall costs are far less when a chiropractor is consulted.

If you have any type of pain, especially pain in the face and head, consult a chiropractor. He'll probably work with an orofacial pain specialist.

Craniosacral Therapy

Craniosacral therapy is a very gentle, non-invasive therapy that focuses on the bones of the skull (cranium) and the sacrum or tailbone. Anyone studying anatomy is told the bones of the skull fuse together by the end of puberty. However, I was curious enough to question this centuries-old concept, and with a microscope, I examined the histology of junctions of several cranial bones. I couldn't believe my eyes. The bones didn't fuse because periosteum (the outside covering of bone) was present, covering each bone at the suture or junction of the bones. To me, this proved the cranial bone didn't fuse, thus movement was not only possible, but likely with the cranial bones.

The movement of cranial bones can be restricted by trauma to the head, pushing on the head (for example, pushing on the skull while sleeping), clenching, or using a TMJ splint which tightly binds the upper teeth, thus preventing the movement of the maxillary bones and subsequently, other bones which articulate (connect to) the maxillary bones.

The craniosacral system consists of the cranial bones, the membranes (fascia) and cerebrospinal fluid that surround and protect the brain and spinal cord and the bones of the spine. It extends from the bones of the skull, face and mouth -- which make up the cranium -- down to the sacrum, or tailbone.

This form of therapy has been effective in evaluating and treating problems associated with generalized pain and dysfunction, lowered vitality, recurring infections, headaches and facial pain. The light touch employed in this approach encourages your own natural mechanisms to improve the functioning of your brain and spinal cord, to dissipate the negative effects of stress.

In the early 1900s, Dr. William Sutherland first developed a system of examination and treatment for the bones of the skull, but because few knew about Sutherland's craniosacral therapy, and because the results seemed miraculous, his work was discounted. Craniosacral therapy was revitalized by Dr. John Upledger in the early 1970s, and he continues to be the most prominent teacher and practitioner of craniosacral therapy throughout the world.

Acting like a semi-closed hydraulic system, pressures build within the craniosacral system as the amount of cerebrospinal fluid increases. As the fluid moves, bathing the brain and the spinal cord, the membranes containing the fluid move, normally at a rate of 6 to 12 cycles per minute. Through this respiratory mechanism, the bones of the cranium and sacrum also move, allowing for these fluctuations of fluid pressure.

If restrictions prevent this movement, pressures may be exerted on the soft tissue of the membranes, brain and spinal cord. An imbalance in the system can adversely affect the development and function of the brain and spinal cord, which can result in sensory, motor and intellectual dysfunction.

Certain types of orofacial pain and headaches respond well to craniosacral therapy. Dr. Upledger reports an 80 to 85% success rate in treating chronic, severe, and disabling headaches. I've personally relieved all types of facial pain, temporal and occipital headaches using cranial techniques.

> *Certain types of orofacial pain and headaches respond well to craniosacral therapy.*

Many chiropractic physicians, medical massage therapists, osteopathic physicians, and some TMJ dentists use craniosacral therapy in their practices. If you're experiencing orofacial pain, find a therapist who uses this gentle technique. If you're wearing a TMJ splint on your upper teeth which is tightly bound to the teeth, I guarantee you'll have cranial bone restriction. Many times, just by changing the splint or making an existing one fit more loosely, I've been able to stop facial and headache pain.

Like chiropractic, craniosacral therapy offers another effective, alternative mode of therapy for orofacial pain.

Medical Massage Therapy

Massage is among the oldest of all medical treatments used by man. Records indicate that ancient Hindus, Persians and Egyptians used forms of massage for some ailments, and Hippocrates (in the 5th century B.C.) wrote papers recommending the use of rubbing and friction for joint and circulation problems.

Today, massage is an accepted part of many physical rehabilitation programs and has proven beneficial for many chronic conditions such as low back pain, arthritis and bursitis, head and facial pain. Massage helps relieve the stress and tension stored in muscles in the form of trigger points, or areas of chronic contraction, producing pain and dysfunction.

We prescribe massage therapy for its soothing, healing and recuperative benefits. It's useful for restoring muscles to their normal function by breaking spasms and tightness caused by prolonged postural positions (i.e., trigger points). Massage is instrumental in healing "pulled," strained or overused muscles and tendons. The effects of a common orofacial pain problem easily treated by massage is bruxism. Chronic clenching and/or grinding of the teeth quickly fatigues the muscles which move the mandible. Massage relieves the trigger points which develop in these muscles and reduces the patient's overall stress.

Today, most states license medical massage therapists (also called massotherapists). These therapists are fast becoming a integral part of the health care team. Also, many chiropractic physicians work hand in hand with massage therapists, oftentimes within the same office.

Under the title Massage Therapy, therapists use several forms or variations built upon the five basic strokes of Swedish massage:

- **Effleurage:** Slow, rhythmic, gliding strokes, usually in the direction of blood flow toward the heart. Usually the massage therapist uses the whole hand (palm and fingers), gradually applying an increasing amount of pressure. Variations of effleurage involve strokes applied with the fingertips, heel of the hand, or knuckles.

- **Petrissage:** Kneading, pressing, and rolling muscle groups. The massage therapist holds the tissue and alternately tightens and loosens his grasp.

- **Friction:** Steady pressure or tight circular movements across muscle fibers without moving across the skin, often used in areas around joints.

- **Percussion:** Drumming hand movements on broad areas of the body, particularly the back. Techniques include beating with the side of loosely clenched fists; cupping or striking with the fingertips and heel of the hand; hacking, rapid chopping motions with the edge of the hand; and clapping, using the flattened hand to clap rapidly over fleshy areas.

- **Vibration and Jostling:** Vibration entails rapid movements by the therapist to transmit an oscillating action to the patient. Mechanical vibrators are also used for this purpose.

Jostling requires rapid shaking of a muscle back and forth, usually for a brief period.

You might also encounter some specialized techniques employed for specific purposes. These include:

- **Neuromuscular Massage:** Also known as trigger point therapy, this technique applies concentrated finger pressure to painful areas in muscles called trigger points. This is probably the most useful form of massage therapy for treating orofacial and headache pain. I often teach my patient's spouse to perform a variation of this technique, thereby getting the spouse involved, which helps the patient physically and both spouses emotionally.

- **Deep Tissue Massage:** The use of slow strokes and deep finger pressure on areas of the body suffering from chronic muscle tension or areas that simply ache or feel contracted. Deep tissue massage is especially effective with tense areas such as stiff necks or sore shoulders, both of which refer pain directly into the face and temples.

- **Sports Massage:** This rapidly expanding field, popular among both professional athletes and fitness enthusiasts, focuses on the use of massage to assist training, prevent injury, and aid healing in case of soreness or injury. It's used both before and after exercise, as well as in the treatment of sports injuries such as sprains, strains, and tendinitis.

- **Manual Lymph Drainage:** This rhythmic pumping form of massage stimulates the movement of lymph fluid through the lymph vessels. It is used to treat edema, or an accumulation of lymph, producing tissue swelling.

How do you find a medical massage therapist? Ask your doctor, chiropractor, or look in directories for therapists who are members of the American Massage Therapy Association (AMTA). Membership means the therapist has graduated from a training program approved by the Commission on Massage Training Accreditation/Approval, holds a state license that meets AMTA certification standards, has passed an AMTA membership examination, or has passed the National Certification Examination for Therapeutic Massage and Bodywork.

Neural Therapy

Neural therapy may also be helpful in treating orofacial pain. This unique type of therapy uses injections of local anesthetic to remove short circuits in the body's electrical network. In theory, this frees up the body's flow of energy and normalizes cellular function.

In 1928, two German physicians and brothers, Ferdinand and Walter Huneke, introduced neural therapy to medicine. They discovered that by injecting procaine (the true Novocaine) into nerves of the autonomic nervous system, scars, and glands, pain and autonomic dysfunction were often relieved permanently. At times, a series of injections are required, but other times, just one injection is sufficient.

According to the brothers Huneke and current proponents of neural therapy, neural theory actually works at the biological energy level. Everything alive is electrically charged, and each cell has its own specific frequency range. As long as the energy flowing throughout the body is within its normal frequency range, the tissues will remain healthy.

Injuries and chronic illnesses are caused (according to neural theory) by changes or interferences in the normal electrical conductivity of cells and of the autonomic nerves. This interruption of the normal electrical flow creates an interference field, interfering with normal health of the tissues, thus producing disease, pain, and dysfunction.

The local anesthetic (neural-therapeutic agent) injected into the interference field has a high electrical potential of its own which restores and stabilizes the defective cell membrane electrical potential. The "error" or interference of the autonomic nervous system is corrected, at least temporarily, restoring the normal electrical flow. Each repetitive injection improves the tissue's ability to recharge and maintain the necessary and healthy electrical potential.

Neural therapy is used by many practitioners to treat all types of orofacial and TMJ pain. Usually, the facial ganglion (collection of nerve cells) and various trigeminal nerve branches are injected with procaine. Also, scars, which create an interference field and may generate pain, respond well to neural therapy injections.

Acupuncture

Acupuncture originated in China well over five thousand years ago. It was brought to the United States in the mid 1800s, but it was largely ignored in America until the early 1970s. Although practitioners of acupuncture claim it's useful for all types of maladies, the Western world's interest in this ancient art has chiefly been in pain relief.

According to the Chinese Pain Center in Hacienda Heights, California, acupuncture is a method of encouraging the body to promote natural healing and to improve functioning. This is done by inserting needles and applying heat or electrical stimulation at very precise acupuncture points. Moxibustion, the warming of acupuncture points through the use of herbal applications, is often used as a supplement, and the needles may also be stimulated using a small electric current.

The classical Chinese explanation is that channels of energy run in regular patterns through the body and over its surface. These channels, called meridians, are supposedly like rivers flowing through the body to irrigate and nourish the tissues. Blood flow and nerve impulses also follow meridians to run through the body to various parts, structures and organs. An obstruction in the movement of these energy rivers is like a dam that backs up the flow in one part of the body and restricts it in others. Any obstruction and blockages or deficiencies of energy, blood and nerve impulses eventually lead to disease.

The meridians are influenced by needling the acupuncture points: The acupuncture needles unblock the obstruction at the dams, and reestablish the regular flow through the medians. Acupuncturists claim treatments help the body's internal organs to correct imbalances in their digestion, absorption, and energy production activities, and in the circulation of their energy through the meridians.

In short, in traditional Chinese medicine, Yin represents "-" (negative) and Yang represents "+" (positive). The main principle of Chinese medicine is to keep the Yin and Yang balance or bring Yin and Yang back into balance. Yin -- Yang balanced is the healthy state of the body. Needling acupuncture points, tp re-establish the regular flow through the meridians, balances Yin and Yang.

The modern, generalized scientific explanation is that needling the acupuncture points stimulates the nervous system to release chemicals (endorphins and enkephlins) in the muscles, spinal cord, and brain. These chemicals will either change the experience of pain, or they'll trigger the release of other chemicals and hormones which influence the body's own internal regulating system. The improved energy and biochemical balance produced by acupuncture stimulates the body's natural healing abilities, and apparently, promotes physical and emotional well-being. Using a TENS unit (Transcutaneous Electrical Nerve Stimulator) works in a similar fashion by causing endorphin release.

Proponents of acupuncture also explain the physics of this ancient healing art on a cellular and molecular level. The very basic unit of the body is cell. According to proponents of acupuncture, the movement of cells follows the movement of electrons. The electrons inside cells act according to their own regular patterns. These electrons in the body are termed bioelectrons.

Energy flow in the meridians is the direct or indirect transportation of bioelectrons. Meridians are the pathways where bioelectrons move through the body. When positive and negative charges in the bioelectronic movements are not balanced, the cells act abnormally -- This is Yin and Yang imbalance. In Chinese medicine, this imbalance is defined as disease. It's a beginning stage of the physiological cells electrons movement. The Chinese believe only radical change of the cells' electron movement is admitted by Western medicine.

All the external factors, such as mechanical, physical, chemical, biological influences and internal factors such as mental, hereditary, constitutional influences cause an imbalance in the body's bioelectrical movement, leading to disease.

Apparently, acupuncture may force the bioelectrons to resume their normal and regular movement patterns, thus restoring the Yin -- Yang balance. The more acupuncture treatments the patient has, the longer the normal movement pattern of the bioelectrons remains until finally the electrons inside cells don't follow the abnormal movement pattern any further. At this point, the problem is considered solved.

Acupuncture seems to also be effective in providing local anesthesia. I had a good friend who was severely wounded in Vietnam, and underwent spinal surgery, with acupuncture the only type of anesthesia provided. Colleagues have witnessed major abdominal surgeries, again with acupuncture being the only type of anesthesia offered.

Most of us in traditional medicine think of acupuncture only as being helpful in the relief of pain. However, acupuncturists believe it's also effective in treating a wide variety of conditions through its power to stimulate the mind and body's own healing response.

During acupuncture treatment, needles (usually made from gold) are either inserted for a second or two or left in place for up to 20 to 30 minutes, depending on the effect required. During this time, some patients report a heavy sensation in the limbs and a pleasant feeling of relaxation.

Sometimes, an herbal preparation (known as a moxa) is applied over, or held near, the acupuncture point and removed when the patient feels it becoming hot. Gentle electrical stimuli may also be applied through the needles, giving a sensation of tingling or buzzing.

Other methods of treating acupuncture points include massage (acupressure), tapping with a rounded probe, and laser therapy at acupuncture points. These are techniques that are particularly suitable for children or for people who have a genuine fear of needles.

Treatment with acupuncture can produce rapid results, but more often it requires a number of treatments over a period of time. Usually treatments are once or twice a week, but they can be less frequent. Sometimes the effect is dramatic, and the patient will only need one or two treatments. In other cases, the effect is subtle, and one may require treatment for several months.

Does acupuncture really work? Look at the results of a survey of 575 participants, conducted by Claire Cassidy, Ph.D. According to her, this is the largest survey to date of acupuncture patients.

- 91.5% reported "disappearance" or "improvement" of symptoms after treatment

- 84% reported they consulted their traditional doctors less

- 58.5% said they were seeing a psychotherapist less

- 78.9% reported they used fewer prescription medications

- 77.5% saw their physical therapist less

- 70.1% of those whom surgery have been recommended said they avoided it

Understandably, this population of 575 patients was not a random sample, as they all had been treated with acupuncture and, obviously, supported this type of alternative therapy. However, these statistical numbers would be impressive even if they were cut in half.

A Personal note. I've had a few hours of training in acupuncture through the American Academy of Pain Medicine. In fact, being the curious person I am, I volunteered to be used as an example demonstrating the proper placement of acupuncture needles. The lecturer attempted to relieve my lower back pain.

Inserting the needles (in my ears, ear lobes and hand) was virtually painless, but when they were twirled, I felt a tingling and a couple of times, a bright, shooting, electrical type of sensation (similar to what you might experience when your dentist gives you an anesthetic injection to numb your lower jaw). After a few minutes, I felt a tingling all around the needles . . .even some itching. The needles were left in place about 20 or 25 minutes. I didn't receive any back pain relief, but to be honest, one treatment rarely (as I understand it) produces pain relief.

Would I recommend acupuncture for my orofacial pain patients? Maybe, but not as the first course of therapy. Would I be opposed to a patient seeking treatment from an acupuncturist? Certainly not. I believe acupuncture, like other forms of alternative therapy, provides one more avenue to pursue for doctors and patients alike in the quest to conquer chronic pain.

I guess East is meeting West, but personally, I'll take a traditional, allopathic general anesthesia if my gall bladder ever needs to be removed!

Vitamin Therapy

Probably the most controversial area in medicine today is the validity of vitamin therapy. Like most doctors except chiropractics and naturopathic physicians, I was trained in traditional or allopathic nutrition. Although we had excellent training in biochemistry and physiology, our nutritional training was sadly lacking. It consisted of the four basic food groups and how we might counsel our patients in the prevention of tooth decay and periodontal disease. There was never any real attention paid to true body chemistry. In fact, the concept of nutrition was scoffed at. Medical science was far too advanced to worry about such trivial items as cellular metabolism, proper supplementation and so forth. Modern medicine had all the answers, and besides, if we or our patients became ill, we'd just write a prescription, and everything would be alright. Usually. Regardless if you have orofacial pain or not, the scientific evidence, which is overwhelming and continues to grow, recommends we all take a minimum daily dosage of specific vitamins. Michael Murray, N.D., in his authoritative and comprehensive book, *Encyclopedia of Nutritional Supplements*, recommends the following:

• Take a high quality vitamin and mineral supplement. The sad truth is you get what you pay for, generally. I've seen an interesting plaque which reads, "Don't take chances with parachute packers or your health."

- Take extra antioxidants. Hardly a week passes that the press doesn't report another scientific study which recommends the use of antioxidants. Science is finally catching up with naturopathy.

- Take one tablespoon of flaxseed oil daily. This natural oil is an excellent source of omega 3 fatty acids, which, among other benefits, reduces the production of arachidonic acid, the precursor of many inflammatory products which are the chief causes of inflammation and localized pain.

In my practice, I recommend vitamin and mineral therapy (collectively termed supplements) for all my patients who suffer with facial pain, and especially for those who require any type of surgery. I can't express how important these supplements are and how quickly surgical patients, for example, heal compared to those who don't take supplements.

Table 13.1 lists the common supplements which I prescribe for many of my patients. I provide them or insist the patients go to a health food store to ensure they'll purchase quality supplements.

Obviously, other minerals (e.g., manganese, chromium and others) are important and you need to consider taking

Table 13.1: Suggested supplements and dosages.

Supplement	Suggested Daily Dosage	Comments
Calcium	2,000 mg	For proper muscular function and calming; prevents bone decalcification and relieves stress. Used chelated forms.
Magnesium	1,500 mg in divided dosages	For proper muscle function
Vitamin B Complex	100 mg 3 times per day	Provides all the benefits of the B vitamins (e.g., antioxidant)
Vitamin C	1,000 mg 2 to 5 times per day	Coenzyme in production and repair of connective tissues; antioxidant.
Coenzyme Q10	100 mg	Improves oxygenation of tissues
Vitamin E	400 IU 2 to 3 times per day	Antioxidant; protects red blood cells; essential in cellular respiration
Multivitamins & Minerals	As directed	For balanced nutrition.

these as well. I'd suggest consulting a good book on nutrition, such as Dr. Michael Murray's book, *Encyclopedia of Nutritional Supplements.*

Herbal Medicine

Herbs have been used for centuries. Records of the Romans, Egyptians, Persians and Native Americans are filled with accounts of the extensive use of herbs to treat all types of diseases, including pain. Today, approximately one-third of prescription medicines are derived from plants.

Herbs usually are gentler and safer than prescription drugs. They also produce less side effects, but they may be harmful if taken improperly or in excess. It's best to consult a health care practitioner who is trained in herbology.

Herbs are used in several ways, such as:

- **Compresses.** A compress is a cloth soaked in an herbal solution and applied directly on the painful area of the body.

- **Decoctions.** A decoction is a tea which contains an herb.

- **Essential oils.** Usually mixed with vegetable oil or water, essential oils may be used as mouthwashes, an inhalant, a tea drink, or rubbed externally on painful areas.

- **Extracts.** The most effective form of herbal preparations, extracts are prepared by pressing herbs with hydraulic pressure and soaking them in alcohol or water. The excess liquid is permitted to evaporate, leaving a strong extract.

You can find herbs in the form of teas, capsules, tablets, beverages, creams, tinctures, lotions, powders and oils. In most cases, the bitter-tasting herbs are the medicinal ones. Don't use herbs for extended periods of time.

Some of the more common herbs you might try for orofacial pain are:

- **Aloe vera.** Aloe vera is very soothing for skin irritations and open cuts and abrasions. Try this herb to combat the pain of herpes zoster. I've had good success by recommending that my patients crush an aspirin and mix it with aloe vera to be used as a salve. You might also try mixing cayenne pepper with aloe vera as a salve.

- **Arnica.** This herb reduces pain by soothing the nerves. You can take arnica as a tea, or use it as a compress, or apply it as an oil.

- **Cayenne pepper.** A favorite herb in Mexican food, cayenne pepper has recently gained great acceptance in the world of traditional medicine as a strong pain killer. Actually, it's the capsaicin in the pepper which prevents the production of the powerful pain neurotransmitter Substance P.

- **Chamomile.** Chamomile is effective against inflammation, and it produces mild sedation and relieves muscle spasms. Many use it for facial pain, especially pain from neuralgia. Take chamomile as a tea or as a compress.

- **Feverfew.** Recently feverfew has been gaining fame as a effective treatment for migraine headaches. It also helps ease diseases caused by chronic inflammation such as arthritis by inhibiting the release of two inflammatory substances, serotonin and prostaglandins.

- **Ginger.** Like chamomile and wintergreen (see below), ginger works well against inflammation and pain. It works best in capsule form.

- **Goldenseal.** This herb is reportedly a good anti-inflammatory one, although this is not its primary action.

- **Horehound.** Good for sinusitis (but honestly, I'd rather have the disease than taste this stuff!).

- **Kava kava.** Kava kava has been used for over 3,000 years for its medicinal effects as a sedative and muscle relaxant.

- **Melatonin.** In the early 1990s, melatonin became a popular supplement for counteracting jet lag and helping people sleep. I often recommend that a patient use melatonin to improve the quality of sleep before a prescription medication.

- **Skullcap.** A good sedative.

- **St. John's Wort.** Historically used as a nerve tonic, St. John's wort is now widely used as a mild antidepressant because it works as a serotonin reuptake inhibitor, just like the tricyclic antidepressants drugs (e.g., Nortriptyline). It's also helpful in reducing one's perception of pain. The most well known action of St. John's wort is in repairing nerve damage and reducing pain and inflammation.

- **Valerian.** Also a good sedative.

- **Wild yam.** Reduces inflammation and relaxes muscle spasms.

- **Wintergreen.** Wintergreen contains salicylate, the active ingredient in aspirin. It's helps reduce inflammation and swelling and used topically, not orally.

Tai Chi

Tai Chi (pronounced Tie Chee) is an ancient form of martial arts, developed in China well over 1,000 years ago. Through Tai Chi, the Chinese attempted to combine both physical and mental conditioning to restore order in one's body and mind. Unlike other martial art forms (e.g., karate), Tai Chi is a series of gentle exercises designed to bring balance and harmony to the body and mind, which, in turn, allow the "life-force" of chi to flow.

The Chinese believe chi is the force of life. They believe this force, flowing freely through the body, is essential for a healthy life. Because chi is blocked by stress (according to the theory) and since stress is a major perpetuating factor of chronic pain, the slow and gentle movements of Tai Chi supposedly reduce stress and restore this free-flowing force with relaxation. Proponents of Tai Chi believe this relaxation technique basically dissipates mental stress by:

- Relaxing the mind through slow, flowing movements, reducing physical stress

- Removing the physical overall effects of stress

Tai Chi practitioners combine slow, deliberate and circular movements, meditation and deep breathing to quiet the body and mind with relaxation and renewed chi.

A *Personal note.* Although I don't agree with much of the Chinese metaphysical philosophy of chi nor do I participate in meditation (except of the Word of the Lord [Psalm 1:2 and Psalm 143:5]), as a martial artist, I practice Tai Chi. My sensei (teacher) and I talk for hours about Eastern philosophy and the Christian faith, especially concerning we as marital artists. He's patient with me, and I'm firm with him. Yin and Yang perhaps?

Regardless of one's philosophy, I recommend this gentle activity for my orofacial pain patients as it's a slow, smooth method of obtaining physical activity and reducing both physical and mental stress.

Magnet Therapy

Using magnets to improve health has recently gained great momentum in the circles of alternative treatments. However, this controversial, yet safe form of therapy has been used for centuries. Proponents of magnetotherapy, as this type of treatment is known, use magnets for the treatment of virtually every ailment, including chronic pain. In 1978, the U.S. Food and Drug Administration approved the use of magnets for general purposes as a non-invasive mode of therapy.

How does magnetotherapy work to reduce pain and cure diseases? First, it's important to know there are channels in cells termed voltage gated ionic channels. The opening and closing of these tiny channels are regulated by electrical charges. Certain conditions produce opening or closing of these channels, permitting the movement of molecules and ions (electrically charged atoms) through them. Some researchers feel magnets act like regulators by changing the electrical charge of the cells in the magnetic field. It also seems that magnetotherapy may causes changes in molecular shapes, changes in blood flow, and actually drive certain nutrients into cells, all of which supposedly produces a healing effect. According to practitioners of magnetotherapy, pain is reduced because the change in electrical charge generated by using magnets tends to drive oxygen molecules through the ion channels, improving the chemical environment of the cells.

How far does magnetotherapy penetrate the body? Some studies show the penetration depth may be up to 30 inches, far deeper than ultrasound or electrical stimulation. So, theoretically, magnets can used for superficial and deep illnesses and pain. Those who recommend magnetotherapy apply the negative (North Pole) magnet directly over the painful area. Consult an alternative therapist for more information.

Aromatherapy

Aromatherapy uses pure essential oils, extracted from many parts of the plant (flower, leaf, resin, bark, root, twig, seed, berry, rind and rhizome) to relax, balance and rejuvenate body, mind and spirit. Aromatherapy is both an art and a science.

Essential oils, as implied by the term aromatherapy, have a powerful effect through our sense of smell. Simply by inhalation, essential oils elicit an immediate olfactory response, and they are readily absorbed into the bloodstream

The results of aromatherapy are very individual. While there is general agreement about the actions of certain oils, aromatherapy texts vary in their descriptions of the properties and characteristics of an essential oil. No two persons are affected by the same essential oil in exactly the same way. Even the same person can be affected differently by the same oil depending on surroundings, time of day or mood, or so the theory goes.

Aromatic medicine, the ancient beginnings of today's art of aromatherapy, was recorded in both Egypt and India more than 4,500 years ago. The Egyptians used aromatic plants to create massage oils, medicines, embalming preparations, skin care products, fragrant perfumes and cosmetics. Plant aromatics were also utilized in India as part of the ancient medical practice known as Ayurveda. Many of these practices are still in existence today.

In 3000 B.C. in China, Emperor Huang Ti included aromatherapy in his book on internal medicine. Hippocrates described the effects of over 300 plants for medicinal purposes.

In 900 A.D., Avicenna the Arabian physician (the same Avicenna who also wrote about trigeminal neuralgia) wrote several books on the properties of plants and made a significant contribution to the distillation process of oils from plants by improving the cooling system.

At the beginning of this century, particularly in France and England, a movement by noted doctors and scholars in the naturopathic and medical communities prompted a reawakening to the benefits of natural medicine and aromatherapy. The actual term aromatherapy was coined by Rene Gattefosse, a French chemist, in the 1920s. He investigated the antiseptic properties of essential oils and discovered the healing properties of lavender. His book, Aromatherapie, was published in 1928.

Today in England and the United States, aromatherapy is becoming an accepted alternative medicine. In France, it is common to find doctors who practice aromatherapy, pharmacies that sell essential oils and health insurance companies that reimburse for treatments using these approaches.

Essential oils are the highly concentrated, volatile, aromatic essences of plants. Scientists agree that essential oils may perform more than one function in living plants. In some cases they seem to be a part of the plant's immune system. In other cases they may simply be end-products of metabolism. Essential oils contain hundreds of organic constituents, including hormones, vitamins and other natural elements that work on many levels. They are 75 to 100 times more concentrated than the oils in dried herbs.

All the countries of the world provide essential oils, making aromatherapy a truly global therapy. The purest essential oils come from carefully cultivated and wild grown plants from climatic and geographic regions throughout the world.

Essential oils absorb into the fluid surrounding the cells beneath the skin's surface for a variety of effects including deep cleansing, nourishing, rejuvenating and balancing. Essential oils also diffuse into the air to provide olfactory benefits like purifying, refreshing and relaxing.

Essential oils are the foundation on which aromatherapy is built. Essential oils fall into several basic categories:

1. **Monoterpenes:** anti-viral, antiseptic, bactericidal, and can be highly irritating to the skin. Examples: lemon, pine, frankincense.

2. **Esters:** fungicidal, sedating, and very aromatically pleasing. Examples: bergamot, clary sage, lavender.

3. **Aldehydes:** sedating and antiseptic. Examples: melissa, lemongrass, citronella.

4. **Ketones:** ease congestion, aid flow of mucus, can be toxic. Examples: fennel, hyssop, sage.

5. **Alcohols:** very antiseptic, anti-viral with uplifting qualities. Examples: rosewood, geranium, rose.

6. **Phenols:** bactericidal and strongly stimulating, can be highly irritating to the skin. Examples: clove, thyme, oregano.

7. **Oxides:** expectorant and bactericidal. Examples: rosemary, tea tree.

Aromatherapy is often combined with massage therapy, but benefits from essential oils are also reported from baths, inhalation, vaporization and gargling.

How scientific is aromatherapy? That's a good question. However, recently, at Queen's Hospital in Birmingham, England, jasmine was shown to dramatically reduce the effects of epilepsy in one patient. All unconscious, dysfunctional electrical discharges of the brain, which occurred every 10 seconds totally stopped after a patient was administered aromatherapy using jasmine only two times. This is interesting and should encourage more research on this subject.

Table 13.2: Essential oils used to treat orofacial pain.		
Disorder	**Primary Essential Oil**	**Secondary Oil**
Anxiety	Basil Bergamot Clary-sage Thyme	Chamomile Geranium Juniper Lavender Marjoram Melissa
Headache	Basil Lemon	Aniseed Chamomile Lavender Marjoram Melissa Peppermint Rosemary
Sinus Pain	Basil Lemon Eucalyptus	Lavender Peppermint Pine
Neuralgia	Eucalyptus	Camphor Hyssop
Muscle Pain	Eucalyptus Sage Thyme Cajuput Lavender Caraway	Camphor Chamomile Juniper Majoram Rosemary
Muscle Sprains	Eucalyptus	Camphor Hyssop
Insomnia	Basil Thyme	Camphor Chamomile
Mouth Ulcers	Tea Tree Oil	Thyme Sage
Swelling	Petitgrain	Geranium Juniper

Disclaimer

In all my years of practice, I've never met a colleague, regardless of his or her degree or speciality, who wasn't totally dedicated to relieving pain and suffering. However, I've also met many colleagues, especially many who use various techniques of Alternative Medicine, who were deeply involved in the New Age movement . To my horror, some have been openly involved in the occult through some of the perverted teachings which have infiltrated Alternative Medicine. As a Christian, I must be cautious concerning these attitudes, which are totally contrary to the Christian faith.

Most doctors and therapists wish to do nothing but help their patients, no matter what methods or techniques are required. This is the problem: Some of these well-meaning people use techniques which, as a Christian, I can't nor will not endorse or practice. This doesn't mean these techniques don't work, but from where does the ultimate power arise?

Many who read this book will be upset with my convictions, but I don't have to please anyone but the Lord. When I feel uncomfortable about a certain aspect of alternative medicine, I do as the Apostle John suggested and "test the spirits." (I Jn 4:1)

I'm not indicting or even implying anything negative against those who practice Alternative Medicine. I use many of these techniques myself, yet I constantly remember the verse, "But as for me and my house, we will serve the Lord." (Jos 24:15)

References

1. **Alix ME, Bates DK:** *A proposed etiology of cervicogenic headache: the neurophysiologic basis and anatomic relationship between the dura mater and the rectus posterior capitis minor muscle.* J Manipulative Physiol Ther 1999;22:534-539.

2. **Balch, J. and Balch, P.** *Prescription for Nutritional Healing, 2nd ed.* Golden City Park (NY): Avery Publishing Group, 1997.

3. **Comunetti A, Laage S, Schiessl N, Kistler A:** *Characterization of human skin conductance at acupuncture points.* Experientia 1995;51:328-331.

4. **Dundee JW, Ghaly G:** Local anesthesia blocks the antiemetic action of P6 acupuncture. Clinical pharmacology and acupuncture therapeutics 1991;50:78-80.

5. **Fargas-Babjak AM, Poneranz B, Rooney PJ:** *Acupuncture-like stimulation with codetron for rehabilitation of patients with chronic pain syndrome and osteoarthritis.* Acupunct Electro Therap Res 1992;17:95-105.

6. *Alternative Medicine: The Definitive Guide.* **Goldberg B** (ed). Fife (Washington): Future Medicine Publishing, 1995.

7. **Khalsa DS, Stauth C.** *The Pain Cure.* New York: Warner Books, 1999.

8. **Tai Chi Qigong. Khor G. Torrance (CA):** Heian International, 1993.

9. **Meade TW, Dyer S, Browne W, Townsend J, Frank AO:** *Low back pain of mechanical origin.* Brit Med J 1990;300:1431-1437.

10. **Murray M.** *Encyclopedia of Nutritional Supplements: The Essential Guide for Improving Your Health Naturally.* Rocklin (CA): Prima Publishing, 1996.

11. **Jaffe, L.F:** *Electrophoresis along cell membranes.* Nature 1977;265: 600-602.

12. **Johansson A, Wenneberg B, Haraldson T:** *Acupuncture in treatment of facial muscular pain.* Acta Odontolo Scand 1991;49:153-158.

13. **Rubin P:** *Therapeutic acupuncture: a selective review.* South Med J 1977;70: 974-977.

14. **Vernon HT:** *The effectiveness of chiropractic manipulation in the treatment of headache: an exploration in the literature.* J Manipulative Physiol Ther 1995;18:611-17.

15. *Discovery of Magnetic Health.* **Washnis GJ, Hricak RZ.** Rockville: Nova Publishing Co, 1993.

16. *The Complete Book of Homeopathy.* **Weiner M.** Garden City Park: Avery Publishing Group, 1989.

CHAPTER Fourteen

TMJ

WHAT IS TMJ?

Many people, even doctors, nurses, and insurance companies, use the term TMJ. But what does this abbreviation mean?

The term TMJ is an abbreviation for Temporo-Mandibular Joint, or the jaw joint. In fact, there are really two TMJs, one in front of each ear. The TMJ is the joint formed by the temporal bone of the skull (Temporo) with the lower jaw or mandible (hence, mandibular). These joints move each time we chew, talk or even swallow. Therefore, they are probably the most used joints in the body (for some, used far more than in others!).

To accommodate this frequent use and to help us open our mouths wide, the TMJ is actually a sliding joint and not a ball-and-socket like the shoulder. This sliding allows for pressures placed on the joint to be distributed throughout the joint and not just in one area.

In the medical community, the term TMJ is really not correct. It designates an anatomical structure (the TemporoMandibular Joint) and not a painful condition. The correct term, as recommended by the American Dental Association, is TMD, or TemporoMandibular Disorders, a more precise term than TMJ.

> *In the medical community, the term TMJ is really not correct.*

However, in this chapter, TMJ will be used because it is so well known. So when we say TMJ, let's agree that we are talking about a condition that is often quite painful, debilitating, and frustrating.

But the question of what is the condition of TMJ has not been answered. In the strictest sense, TMJ is a set of separate and yet related disorders of the temporomandibular joints and associated structures like muscles, ligaments, tendons, nerves and blood vessels. Traditionally, TMJ was considered to be one problem; today we know that TMJ really means a group of several disorders that usually have similar symptoms. That is one of the main reasons why so many people continue to suffer from a TMJ disorder even though they are being treated by honest, well-meaning practitioners.

TMJ Anatomy

The temporomandibular joint is the most complex joint in the human body. It's formed by the articulation (connection) of the lower jaw or mandible with the upper jaw or temporal bone. Placed between these two bones is a disc, just like the one between your back bones. This disc is primarily made of cartilage and in the TMJ acts like a third bone. The disc, being attached to a muscle, actually moves with certain movements of the TMJ. (Figure 14.1)

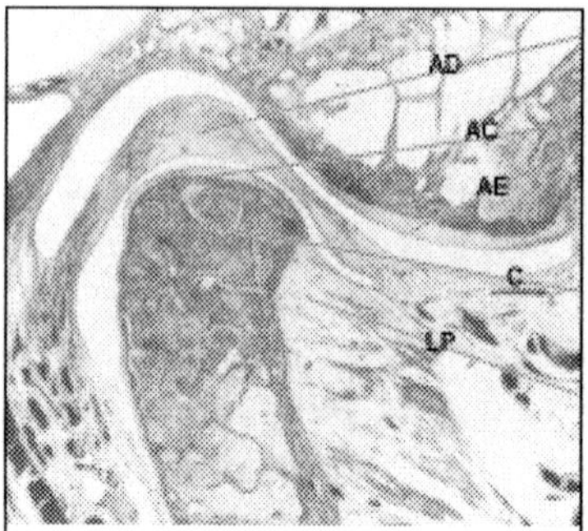

Figure 14.1

AD: Articular disc;
AE: Articular eminence of temporal bond;
LP: Lateral pterygoid muscle;
AC: Artirular cartilage;
C: Condyle of mandible.

The nerve to the TMJ is a branch of the trigeminal nerve (remember trigeminal neuralgia?) and, therefore, an injury to the TMJ may be confused with neuralgia of the trigeminal nerve.

This is important to know: One TMJ can't function without affecting the other one. Put another way, if one TMJ is injured, the other joint will usually become affected sometime in the future. This is true for knees and ankles as well. Injured ligaments rarely completely heal; and this is especially true of those associated with the TMJ. Some of these ligaments of the TMJ are extremely small. Moreover, the forces placed upon them by chewing make it nearly impossible for proper healing to occur.

The two bones of the TMJ are held together by a series of ligaments, any of which can be damaged, just like any other joint. A damaged TMJ ligament usually results in a dislocation of the disc, the lower jaw, or both. Also, the bones are connected by two main muscles: the temporalis, the masseter, and a minor, newly discovered muscle, the zygomandibularis. Any of these muscles may be painful and produce pain in the TMJ or at the very least, abnormal movement of the lower jaw.

Muscles Associated With The TMJ

There are many muscles in the head, neck and face that are associated with the TMJs. In fact, virtually all muscles of the neck, back, throat and face either directly or indirectly affect the TMJs. The primary muscles are termed the muscles of mastication and include the left and right temporalis, lateral and medial pterygoids, and the masseters. These muscles are all controlled by branches of the third division of the trigeminal nerve. The temporalis and masseter muscles close the jaw. They work like the biceps muscle of the arm, drawing the hand up and towards the body. Both the temporalis and masseter are powerful muscles, capable together of applying as much as 185 to 200 pounds of pressure on the teeth. No wonder fillings and cracked teeth can fracture so easily! Its also amazing that the TMJs can withstand over our lifetimes such constant forces. Sometimes they can't.

All of these muscles of mastication are paired: There is one on the right side and one on the left. The temporalis (temple muscle) attaches the entire side of the skull to the lower jaw at a prominent structure termed the coronoid process of the mandible (Figure 3). This powerful muscle closes the mouth and draws the jaw backwards, helping us to chew efficiently. Locate this muscle by lightly pushing against your temple and then clenching your teeth. Feel the slight bulge? That's the anterior belly of the temporalis. When the TMJ is injured or dislocated, it frequently is painful, thus causing a tension headache.

The masseter too, is a powerful muscle and actually gets larger, just like the biceps, if someone clenches or grinds his or her teeth. In concert with the temporalis muscles, the masseter muscles (one on each side) close the lower jaw and aid in chewing. Lightly press your fingers against the sides of your face just below your cheeks, and clench your teeth. Do you will feel the masseters bulge? Often, the masseters become sore after clenching, grinding, or an injury to the TMJ. Also, like the temporalis muscles, the masseters can enlarge like any skeletal muscle when over-used.

The lateral pterygoid muscles are similar to the temporalis and masseter and yet quite different. The lateral pterygoid is composed of two portions or bellies, the superior and inferior. The superior belly is primarily attached to the TMJ's articular disc and is responsible for proper disc movement in coordination with movement of the lower jaw, especially when closing the mouth. By contrast, the inferior belly is predominately attached to the top of the lower jaw (the mandibular condyle) and is accountable for moving the lower jaw forward, thus opening the mouth, and pulling the mandible to one side. This belly works with muscles, known as accessory muscles, located in the throat just under the chin (primarily the mylohyoid, anterior digastric muscles) to open the mouth. Even though these lateral pterygoid bellies work almost in opposition to each other, the same branch of the trigeminal nerve goes to both. Dislocation of the disc of the TMJ produces an increase in muscle tension in both but especially the superior belly. This increased muscle tension can cause pain in the TMJ, the face, the maxillary sinus, or in and behind the eye. Consequently, if your disc is out of place, you may visit an eye doctor or ENT physician due to eye or sinus pain when actually your pain is produced as a result of a displaced TMJ disc.

The fourth muscle of mastication, the medial pterygoid, assists the temporalis and masseter muscles in closing the mouth. This and the masseter muscle form a sling around the back end of the mandible. It runs parallel with the masseter but inside the jaw. Injury to this muscle produces pain in the TMJ, deep in the side of the head, the ear and even the maxillary sinus.

A newly described muscle, the zygomandibularis, should also be included in the group of muscles of mastication. This muscle, which lies right in front of the temporalis, helps to position the condyle up against the articular disc when the mouth closes.

Neck Muscles Associated With the TMJ

The skull and mandible are precariously balanced on the spinal column by a complex series of muscles; and the spinal column is balanced on the pelvis, also by an extensive series of muscles and ligaments. The entire upper body is, in turn, supported by the legs and ultimately the feet. Guess what? This lower body support is also by way of muscles.

Picture a long dining room table with a white table cloth. Perhaps the table is set for Thanksgiving dinner. Imagine pulling slowly but firmly on one corner only. Can you picture a wrinkle formed the entire length of the table cloth? Even though all dishes move, they do so less and less the farther away you move from the area that you pull. Now, picture your head balanced on the spinal column. Can you see how a hip out of place could, just like the table cloth, "wrinkle" the muscles all the way up the back and neck into the head and ultimately, the TMJs? Now you can begin to understand how bad posture, injury to the neck or even the hips can influence the head and TMJs.

We often see patients with their head thrust forward and their chin tilted up. This usually occurs with those who have a small lower jaw or with one who has had a neck injury. This posture also happens in those who sit for hours at a computer or typewriter. Forward head posture causes the mandible to close differently than it should, thus causing malocclusion (bad bite), which in turn may trigger the person to grind or clench his or her teeth. This forward head posture also causes tension in the muscles of the neck and back, producing head, neck and back pain. Frequently, these painful muscles refer pain into the head, face and TMJs, causing both patient and doctor to think that the pain is coming from the TMJs. Can you see how confusing the process of diagnosing pain can be?

The names of the neck and back muscles aren't really important. However, the effect that increased tension in these muscles has is important. If our balance is disturbed for any length of time, we can experience head, neck, facial and TMJ pain without these structures really being physically injured. So you can see that the diagnosis and treatment of pain can be quite complex and misdiagnoses may be common.

SYMPTOMS OF TMJ

Because many different symptoms of TMJ exist, discovering a proper diagnosis can be difficult. However, there are a few classic symptoms which involve the TM joints, ears, head, face and teeth.

TMJs. The most common symptom of TMJ is jaw joint clicking (popping, snapping) or locking. This clicking sound may be so loud that it can be heard by others while you chew. The noise is actually produced by the cartilage disc being caught between the two bones of the TMJ as the lower jaw moves. There may or may not be pain in the joint itself with the sound of a click or pop. But one thing is for sure: If there is a displaced disc, as is usually the case when a click occurs, then the muscles that move the jaw while chewing are more tense than normal. This tenseness can and does cause muscle, facial, head and neck pain.

Locking of the TMJs may be noticed simply by a catching of the lower jaw as it opens. Sometimes, the person with a locked joint must move the jaw to one side or another in order to open wide. Or, a person might have to open until he hears and feels a loud pop, at which point the jaw actually unlocks. As with clicking, there may or may not be pain associated with locking. If the locking is a result of injury to the head or jaw, pain almost always occurs.

A dislocated TMJ may also be noticed by a change in the dental occlusion, or bite. If the TMJ disc goes out of place, the bones and disc do not fit together properly and, therefore, the bite of the teeth changes.

One last comment about a dislocated TMJ disc: The TMJ can actually lock wide open. This is a very terrifying experience. It usually occurs after a wide opening movement such as a yawn. However, an open lock of the TMJ can also occur after a long dental appointment, being put to sleep for any type of surgery, or even after opening wide to eat an apple or large sandwich. If this open locking occurs again and again, it is generally a sign of weak or loose TMJ ligaments. We often see this in teenaged girls who are so limber that they are able to perform as cheerleaders or gymnasts.

EARS. Due to the close relationship of the development of the TMJs and ears, an injury to the TMJ often causes ear symptoms. Some of the symptoms are pain, fullness or stuffiness, and even a loss of hearing. That is why many TMJ sufferers first go to their family doctor and then to an ear doctor for help. Usually, an examination of the ear is normal, even if there appears to be a loss of hearing. Some patients even take several different types of antibiotics because of the fullness in the ears, even in the absence of other symptoms (fever, redness, heat, discharge).

HEAD. Headache is one of the most common symptoms of a TMJ problem. Although any area of the head may be affected, usually the TMJ headache is located in the temples, back of the head, and even the shoulders. Clenching and grinding of the teeth, both of which themselves may be TMJ symptoms, produce muscle pain which can cause headache pain. Also, a displaced disc in the TMJ may cause pain in the joint, which is often referred into the temples, forehead or neck. These headaches are frequently so severe that they are confused and treated (with little success) for migraine headaches or abnormalities in the brain.

If a patient has seen many different doctors and therapists, has taken all types of medication, has tried all sorts of exercises and still the headache pain persists, then a TMJ problem should be highly suspected. These unfortunate patients often have had numerous x-rays, CT Scans and MRI's. No diagnosis is found, and worse yet, they continue to suffer.

FACE. Anatomically, our faces have more nerves than nearly all other areas of our bodies. Psychologically, we as humans are known by our faces. Although we often attempt to hide our true feelings by wearing a disguise, it is virtually impossible to hide the private experience of pain. When we hurt, our faces show pain. Also, pain from the TMJ may be referred to the face even though the TMJ itself does not really hurt. Facial pain may be deep in the face or on the surface in the skin. The skin might even become sensitive to the touch or to air blowing over it. Often a neurologist is seen for this type of pain.

TEETH. A displaced TMJ disc may cause tooth pain. The teeth may become sensitive to temperatures, especially cold. The teeth may also become sensitive because of jaw activities such as clenching of the teeth or grinding of the teeth. Patients often see their dentist with the complaint of pain in the teeth, and usually the doctor can find no cause. Frequently (and very unfortunately), unnecessary root canals and even tooth extractions are performed in an attempt to help a suffering person. What's worse, after these invasive and non-reversible procedures, patients still have their pain, only now it has increased!

OTHER SYMPTOMS. Many other symptoms may be associated with TMJ. Often, pain will be felt in the shoulders and back due to muscle contraction (a condition called myofascial pain dysfunction syndrome, which was discussed in Chapter 10). Dizziness, disorientation and even confusion are also seen in some people who suffer with TMJ.

Depression is common with TMJ. This may be due to the fact that no one really believes there is a problem causing such pain and suffering. Also, plenty of scientific evidence shows that chronic pain patients (which nearly all TMJ patient can claim) have changes in chemicals in the brain (termed neurotransmitters) as a result of the pain. These chemicals can and do produce depression.

Along with depression comes an inability to get a good night's sleep. This may be due to TMJ pain itself or, changes in the brain's neurotransmitter chemicals which produce stimulation even though the TMJ sufferer is asleep. Sufferers usually wake feeling like they never slept, or at least did not sleep well. This lack of sleep not only makes their pain seem worse, but also adds fuel to the fire of depression.

A TMJ patient may also suffer with photophobia, or light sensitivity. A dislocated TMJ may produce pain in and behind the eye, which can cause sensitivity to light. Blurred vision and eye muscle twitching are also common in TMJ patients.

Another common symptom, and one that prompted Dr. Costen in the 1930s to first write about TMJ, is ringing (termed tinnitus) in the ears. This sound may be caused by many different problems (such as, working around loud noises or taking too much aspirin or ibuprofen). Yet, it is one symptom that I personally see in about 60% of all TMJ patients.

WHAT CAUSES TMJ?

Quite understandably, for years dentists felt that malocclusion, or a bad bite, was the chief cause of TMJ. Physical therapists have been taught that muscle problems and poor posture are the cause for TMJ. Nutritionists contend that poor nutrition may be a major contributing factor and medical doctors list stress as the main cause. Guess what? They're all correct! Many problems can contribute to problems within any joint, but one thing is for sure: there are many different causes. At times, only one major cause can be found. At other times, many factors may contribute to the development of a TMJ problem.

Trauma. According to statistics published in the *Journal of the American Dental Association* in 1991, 44% to 99% of TMJ problems are caused by trauma. By trauma, we mean an injury as obvious as a blow to the jaw with a fist or something as subtle as a whiplash injury with direct trauma to the head or jaw. As you will recall, the lower jaw is connected to the upper jaw by a series of ligaments and muscles. Remember that the disc in the TMJ is held in its proper place by tiny, fragile ligaments. A

> *According to statistics published in the Journal of the American Dental Association in 1991, 44% to 99% of TMJ problems are caused by trauma.*

direct blow to the jaw with a fist, baseball bat, or hitting the steering wheel in an accident may drive the lower jaw upwards and back, thus stretching or tearing these tiny ligaments. The frequent result: a dislocated disc producing a TMJ problem.

This same process occurs in other joints. You certainly know someone who has twisted his or her knee or ankle, tearing ligaments producing a joint injury. If ligaments aren't torn after trauma, the joints can at least be bruised. This bruising produces swelling, a change in the bite, and even ear and headache pain. If the swelling is severe and left untreated, the disc may gradually be displaced, and a click may develop.

Opening Too Wide. All joints have limitations to movement and the TMJ is no exception. If you open wide for a long time, or if your mouth is forced wide open, ligaments again may be torn. Swelling and bruising develop, and disc dislocation may occur. For example, if your mouth is open for a long time at the dental office while having a tooth prepared for a crown, the joint can dislocate. This rarely happens without a prior history of trauma; however, it does happen. Also, this type of injury may occur if someone's mouth is opened too wide when they are being put to sleep for surgery. Again, both of these examples are accidental and consequences of the given procedures.

Bruxism. Bruxism as dicussed, is the abnormal grinding of the teeth. Anyone who has had a small child knows that horrible sound of teeth grinding at nighttime--worse than finger nails on the blackboard! If grinding continues or develops later in life, TMJ may develop. Bruxism usually occurs during sleep. That is why so many people do not realize that they are bruxers. Most of us brux at one time or another. But, if this activity continues for any length of time, then symptoms develop. One indication that a person is a bruxer is sore jaw muscles when waking in the morning. Some researchers feel that the constant grinding of the teeth, causing pressure on the TMJs, may injure the ligaments, thus allowing the disc to dislocate. At the very least, bruxism produces muscle pain and sensitive teeth.

A form of bruxism, clenching, may be a cause of TMJ. Clenching may occur at any time. However, it is noticeable most during times of frustration, concentration or stress. Again, some think that the constant pressures applied to the joints from chronic clenching stretch or injure the ligaments, thereby producing a TMJ problem. See Chapter 11 for a detailed discussion of clenching and bruxism.

Malocclusion. One additional cause of TMJ is malocclusion, or a bad bite. Malocclusion may be produced by poor development of the jaws or removal of teeth without replacement. Malocclusion may also be caused by a high dental restoration, a poor fitting denture or partial denture, or a displaced TMJ disc. Malocclusion may be one cause of bruxism: The bite being off, the brain tends to make a person grind his teeth to even the bite, thus reducing the malocclusion. This becomes a vicious cycle: Malocclusion produces bruxism; bruxism produces sore muscles and sensitive teeth; and sore muscles and sensitive teeth can produce malocclusion.

One important comment must be made about malocclusion. Virtually every dentist believes that malocclusion can cause a TMJ problem; but there has never been a scientifically controlled study to prove this concept. It does stand to reason that the joints could be injured by malocclusion. Yet, this has not been proven.

There has been no scientific controlled study to prove that orthodontic treatment produces a TMJ problem.

Orthodontics. Some dentists feel that orthodontic treatment, or braces, might be a cause of TMJ. By moving teeth with orthodontic appliances, malocclusion is produced during treatment. Also, people undergoing orthodontics do report sensitive teeth, pain in the jaw muscles and even bruxism. However, as with malocclusion, there has been no scientific controlled study to prove that orthodontic treatment produces a TMJ problem. I have seen no correlation with orthodontically treated patients and those suffering with TMJ.

Ligament Laxity. We all remember fellow classmates that were double-jointed meaning that they could bend their fingers back really far or they could put one leg behind their head and so on. Many of these kids became cheerleaders or gymnasts because they were so limber. They were not double-jointed; they actually suffered from a problem termed ligament laxity. If you will also recall, most were girls. This is because women have a hormone that is released from their ovaries (relaxin) which helps in the birth of children. If a young or teenaged girl happens to have a little more of this hormone than normal, and if she also put a lot of stress on joints (in such activities as cheerleading and gymnastics), then her ligaments do not preserve the tightness of a joint. If this occurs, then the joint appears to be double or, loose. This definitely can happen to the TMJ's. Ligament laxity is a fairly common problem in active young women who suffer with TMJ (and injuries to other joints).

Stress. Stress has many effects on our bodies: some good and some bad. Stress, being both physical and psychological, produces an increase in certain chemicals in the blood (catecholamines). These chemicals cause tenseness, restlessness, stimulation and an increase in blood pressure. Blood vessels on the surface of the body constrict and skeletal muscles become tight and develop painful regions termed trigger points. All of these physiological changes can produce muscle tightness and pain. These physical changes are good if you need to "fight or flight" when faced with a stressful situation. However, if you are subjected to chronic stress, these physical changes may produce harmful effects. For example, people subjected to chronic stress develop ulcers, diarrhea, tension headaches, muscle tightness and other physical symptoms.

Now, add these changes to an existing TMJ problem, even one that is hardly noticeable, and a very painful situation occurs. It is just like throwing gasoline on an existing fire: The fire is a TMJ problem, and the gasoline is stress. The gasoline causes the fire to flair up and burn widely for a time, but the gas did not produce the fire (or, TMJ), it just made it worse. This is how it appears that stress acts in conjunction with a TMJ problem. Muscles tighten, teeth clench, abnormal pressure is forced against the TMJ disc, and if the ligaments are weak or if the patient is one that has ligament laxity, then the disc may dislocate.

Treatment Of TMJ

The treatment of TMJ has been controversial. Since dentists are the experts of the jaws, teeth, TMJs and other structures in the head, it is natural that they would provide the most care for TMJ. However, chiropractors, medical doctors, physical and medical massage therapists too, contribute to treatment of these disorders. But usually, dentists treat TMJ.

Dentists use a variety of treatment modalities which may be divided into Phase I and Phase II Therapy. The purpose of Phase I Therapy is to eliminate muscle spasms, TMJ swelling and dislocation (if possible), and generally reduce any type of pain. This treatment usually includes the use of splints, exercises, medication, local anesthetic injections, injections of other medications, physical therapy and chiropractic treatment. Phase I treatment is conservative and reversible.

The purpose of Phase II Therapy is to definitively correct any discrepancies, if necessary, between the upper and lower jaws. Phase II Therapy may include adjustment of the dental occlusion, orthodontics, reconstruction of the teeth, surgery, or a combination of some of the above treatments. It is important to note that Phase II Therapy should not be attempted without successful Phase I Therapy modalities.

For a more detailed discussion of TMJ, see my first book, *TMJ: Its Many Faces.* Much of the information in this chapter is excerpted from my book, with permission of my publisher, Anadem.

References

1. *TMJ: Its Many Faces, 2nd ed.* **Shankland WE.** Columbus: Anadem Publishing, 1998.

2. *Management of Temporomandibular Disorders and Occlusion, 4th ed.* **Okeson JP.** St. Louis: CV Mosby Co, 1998.

CHAPTER Fifteen

Finding a Doctor Who Treats Orofacial Pain

Finding a doctor who knows anything about orofacial pain will be more difficult than you'd believe. Certainly, most dentally related problems can be adequately treated by any dentist. But most of the complex orofacial pain syndromes are recognized by few doctors, regardless of his or her degree.

What can you, as the patient and consumer, do to find the proper type of help? How can you be sure the doctor you consult believes or knows anything about orofacial pain? In my opinion, these are some of the reasons why the cost of the treatment of head, TMJ and orofacial pain is so high. By the time you find someone who can treat you effectively, chances are you have seen several doctors with little or no results.

What's the answer? First, understand that medical doctors were taught precious little about the mouth and face. Unfortunately, medical doctors usually diagnose orofacial pain as neuralgia or sinus problems. After the patient doesn't respond to traditional therapy for these disorders, the doctor most likely will refer them to an ENT physician, a neurologist and ultimately, a psychiatrist.

Many oral and maxillofacial surgeons, on the other hand, also deny the devastating effects that many orofacial pain syndromes have on the sufferer. These doctors, who are actually dentists with a residency in surgery after dental school, generally believe in a theory entitled the Psychophysiologic Theory of Pain. This theory, first popularized in 1969, by oral surgeon Dr. Daniel Laskin, maintains that TMJ and orofacial pain problems can be treated with medication and psychological counseling and usually nothing else. This theory also proposes that nearly all TMJ problems are produced by stress in the sufferer's life, and simply the elimination of the stress will eliminate the pain problem. Unfortunately, most oral surgeons are trained with this theory being prominent. Therefore, consulting an oral and maxillofacial surgeon initially may not be wise.

However, many, if not most, general practitioners of dentistry provide much more help or support than do oral surgeons. Again, this is due to the lack of training of oral surgeons in their residencies concerning orofacial pain disorders. This certainly seems odd and sad. If it weren't for a few pioneers in dentistry, the diagnosis and treatment of orofacial pain would be worse than they presently are.

Why such diversity in dentistry? First, we must consider the type of education in dental school. Most professors of dentistry in the United States, Canada and the rest of the Western world don't practice; they teach only, and unfortunately, they teach as they were taught. Therefore, if these well-meaning professors never learned anything about orofacial pain, they couldn't possibly teach dental students or residents.

Second, treatment varies throughout the United States. Although specific treatment modalities are becoming more consistent and recognized, there still is a great diversity. Diversity is not always wrong. In fact, often there are many different ways to treat the same TMJ problem.

Third, even though doctors (dentists, primarily) believe that facial pain disorders exist, they often look only at the temporomandibular joint and not at other structures. This is especially true in the case of Ernest Syndrome, temporal tendinitis, and any other pain syndrome that has nothing anatomically related to the TMJ. These disorders have only in recent years been discovered and described in the scientific literature. Unfortunately, doctors haven't had the opportunity to read all the journal papers because there are so many journals. I estimate that it will take at least one entire generation of dentists for a recognition of these other disorders to be common.

Fourth, many dentists don't treat orofacial pain because of poor insurance coverage. It is amazing that insurance companies will provide benefits for all other areas of the body except the face. Therefore, and due to the headaches (no pun intended!) caused by insurance companies, many doctors simply refuse to treat these problems. As time goes by, these frustrated practitioners forget to even ask patients if they have symptoms of facial pain syndromes. The patient is the true victim of these administrative disputes.

To add insult to injury, insurance companies insist on calling any pain disorder a TMJ problem, regardless if the joint is involved or not. It's ridiculous, especially when insurance people never even examine the patient.

Thus far, I haven't given you the answer as to how to can find a competent doctor. As you can surmise, this is somewhat difficult. However, there are a few guidelines that you should follow.

Questions.

When calling an office to make an appointment, ask the receptionist to give some information about the doctor.

1. **Does he or she treat many orofacial pain patients?** Unfortunately, the doctor may be wonderful and quite knowledgeable but if few facial pain patients are treated in that office, do you really want to seek care there?

2. **From where do the patients come?** Although it is not always true or a requirement, but knowledgeable doctors treating facial pain generally have patients travel vast distances to see them. Again, this doesn't ensure quality or knowledge.

3. **What kind of training has the doctor had and does he or she attend seminars about facial pain and related problems?** Avoid anyone who doesn't keep up to date in any area of medicine, especially orofacial pain.

4. Does the doctor work with other doctors such as chiropractic physicians? This is important; no doctor can be a Lone Ranger and know-it-all. If he or she claims such nonsense, get out of that office!

5. Would the doctor be offended if you asked for another doctor to give you a second opinion? If a doctor is sure of his or her diagnosis and recommended treatment, a second opinion will be welcomed and not rejected.

6. Does the doctor belong to any TMJ or orofacial pain academies? Although membership to such groups isn't mandatory to demonstrate that the doctor has knowledge concerning orofacial pain, most do belong to one or more of the following groups:

a. The American Academy of Craniofacial Pain;

b. The American Equilibration Society; and,

c. The American Academy of Orofacial Pain (formerly, the American Academy of Craniomandibular Disorders).

After you make your appointment, as the doctor interviews you, interview him or her. Unless you're geographically isolated, allow this doctor to treat you only if you trust and can communicate with him or her. Wouldn't you do the same with a mechanic or builder?

Don't engage in treatment until you understand what the risks of treatment and no treatment.

Also, don't engage in treatment until you understand the risks of treatment and no treatment. Not all pain problems need to be treated more agressively than with a soft diet, moist heat and over the counter medications from time to time. Not all knee or elbow injuries are treated. So, why would all orofacial pain problems need treatment as well?

Further, make certain that you understand what treatment the doctor recommends. In fact, ask for a written statement concerning the proposed treatment and cost for the treatment.

Also, ask what time frame the doctor is contemplating and when you might begin to see improvement.

Remember that, even though you must rely upon someone to treat your problem, understand that they are working for you. I know that this is not a traditional way to view health care. Yet, why should these services be different than any other type of service you may need. Don't allow someone to recommend, much less perform, any type of treatment that doesn't sound right. If the doctor makes a recommendation that you don't feel comfortable with, then ask him or her if there are alternatives. Perhaps there will be none; however, that is rare.

■■■■■*Appendix* A

Resources

1. **Wesley E. Shankland, II, DDS, MS, PhD**
    6011 Cleveland Avenue, Columbus, OH 43231
    1-614-794-0033
    Web site: http://www.drshankland.com

2. **American Academy of Craniofacial Pain**
    520 West Pipeline Road, Hurst, TX 76053
    1-800-322-8651
    Web site: http://www.aacfp.org

3. **American Academy of Orofacial Pain**
    19 Mantua Road, Mount Royal, NJ 08061
    1-609-423-3420
    Web site: http://www.aaop.org

4. **American Academy of Pain Management**
    A13947 Mono Way, Suite #A, Sonora, CA 95370
    Web site: http://www.aapainmanage.org

5. **American Academy of Pain Medicine**
    4700 West Lake Avenue, Glenview, IL 60025
    1-847-375-4731
    Web site: http://www.painmed.org

6. **American Academy of Medical Acupuncture**
    5820 Wilshire Blvd, Suite 500, Los Angeles, CA 90036
    Web site: http://www.medicalacupuncture.org

7. **NTI** Web Site: http://www.nti-tss.com

8. **The Chronic Syndrome Support Association**
    One School Street, Suite 403, Arlington, MA 02476
    781-646-6174
    Web site: http://www.shore.net/~cssa

9. **Dr. Devin Starlanyl's Web Site**
   Web site: http://www.sover.net/~devstar

10. **Dr. James Boyd's Web Site**
    http://www.drjimboyd.com

11. **NICO & Chronic Pain Forum**
    http://forums.delphi.com/dir-app/search/
    index.aspmain.asp?searchString=NICO

12. **Trigeminal Neuralgia Association**
    P.O. Box 340, Barnegat Light, NJ 08006
    1-609-361-6250
    Web site: http://www.tna-support.org

13. **USA Fibromyalgia Association**
    Web site: http://www.w2.com/fibro1.html

14. **Fibromyalgia Association of Greater Washington, DC**
    13203 Valley Drive, Woodbridge, VA 22191-1531
    1-703-790-2324
    Web site: http://www.fmagw.org/

15. **National Center for Complementary
    and Alternative Medicine**
    P.O. Box 8218, Silver Spring, Maryland 20907-8218
    1-888-644-6226
    Web site: http://www.nccam.nih.gov

16. **North American Society of Homeopaths**
    T1122 East Pike Street, # 1122, Seattle, WA 98122
    1-206-720-7000

17. **American Chiropractic Association**
    1701 Clarendon Blvd, Arlington, VA 22209
    1-800-986-4636

18. **Face Pain**
    http://www.facepain.com

■ *Appendix* B

Additional Resources Concerning NICO Lesions

1. **Stockton, S. *Beyond Amalgam*, revised edition.**
Clearwater (FL): Power of One Publishing, 2001.
1-800-830-4778.
http://www.healthcarealternatives.net/

2. **Neville BW, Damm, DD, Allen CM, Bouquot JE.**
Oral & Maxillofacial Pathology, 2nd ed.
Philadelphia: WB Saunders Co, 2001.

3. **Bouquot JE, Roberts AM, Person P:** Neuralgia-
inducing cavitational osteonecrosis (NICO):
osteomyelitis in 224 jawbone samples from patients
with facial neuralgias.
Oral Surg Oral Med Oral Pathol 1992;73:307-319.

4. **Shankland WE:** Craniofacial pain syndromes that
mimic temporomandibular joint disorders.
Ann Acad Med Singapore 1995;24:83-112.

5. **Ratner EJ, Person P, Kleinman DJ, et al:**
Jawbone cavities and trigeminal neuralgia and
atypical facial neuralgias.
Oral Surg Oral Med Oral Pathol 1979;48:3-20.

6. **Roberts AM, Person P:** Etiology and treatment of
idiopathic trigeminal neuralgia and atypical facial
neuralgias.
Oral Surg Oral Med Oral Pathol 1979;48:298-308.

7. **Mathis BJ, Oatis GW, Grisius RJ:** Jaw bone cavities
associated with facial pain syndromes: case reports.
Milit Med 1981;146:719-723.

8.   **Ratner EJ, Langer B, Evins ML:** Alveolar
      cavitational osteopathosis – manifestations of an
      infectious process and its implication in the
      causation of chronic pain.
      J Periodontol 1986;57:593-603.

9.   **Segall RO, Del Rio CE:** Cavitational bone defect:
      a diagnostic challenge. J Endo 1991;17:396-400.

10.   **Harris W:** Recent work on trigeminal nerve.
      Lancet 1939;1:1114.

11.   **Bataineh AB, al-Omari MA, Owais AI:** Arsenical
      necrosis of the jaws. Int Endod J 1997;30:283-287.

12.   **Byron MA:** A clinicopathologic review of 2278
      NICO cases. Master's Thesis. Morgantown (WV):
      West Virginia University, 1994.

13.   **Bouquot JE, McMahon RE:** Ischemic osteonecrosis
      of the jaws in 2,023 patients with facial pain.
      J Oral Pathol Med 1996;25:271 (abstract).

14.   **Bouquot JE, McMahon RE:** Neuropathic pain in
      maxillofacial osteonecrosis.
      J Oral Maxillofac Surg 2000;58:1003-1020.

15.   **Wilensky AO:** Osteomyelitis of the jaw.
      Arch Surg 1932;25:215.

16.   **Hankey GT:** Osteomyelitis (necrosis) of the jaws:
      its pathology and treatment. Br Dent J 1938;63:552.

17.   **Bouquot JE, McMahon RE.** Ischemic osteonecrosis
      in facial pain syndromes. Part 1: a review of NICO
      (neuralgia-inducing cavitational osteonecrosis)
      based on experience with more than 2,000 patients.
      Edition 5.3. Morgantown (WV): The Maxillofacial
      Center;1996:1-19.

About the Author

Dr. Wesley Shankland graduated from The Ohio State University with a Bachelor of Science Degree, majoring in biochemistry and zoology. He continued his education and graduated from The Ohio State University College of Dentistry in 1978. In 1993, he returned to graduate school and earned a Master of Science Degree and a Doctor of Philosophy in human anatomy. Dr. Shankland maintains a private practice in Columbus, Ohio, that is limited to the diagnosis and treatment of craniofacial and temporomandibular joint disorders. Dr. Shankland is a Vietnam era veteran, serving as a corpsman in the U.S. Army.

The author of over 90 scientific publications, a manual of head and neck anatomy, and chapters in several textbooks, he is also the author of the best selling book, *TMJ: Its Many Faces*, which is now in its second edition and published by Anadem Publishers.

Dr. Shankland is a Board Member of the American Academy Craniofacial Pain (formerly, the American Academy of Head, Neck and Facial Pain), and has served as the Academy's president from 1998 through 2000. He's also a member of the American Academy of Orofacial Pain, the American Headache Society, The American Equilibration Society, the American Academy of Clinical Anatomists, the American Academy for the Advancement of Science, and the Christian Medical and Dental Society. He's board certified by the American Academy of Head, Neck and Facial Pain, the American Academy of Neurological and Orthopedic Surgery, and the American Academy of Pain Management.

Dr. Shankland has taught courses and given lectures throughout North American, Mexico, the Caribbean, England and Germany concerning orofacial pain, head and neck anatomy, the differential diagnosis of headaches, and temporomandibular disorders. He the Associate Editor of the *Journal of Craniomandibular Practice* and on the editorial boards of three other scientific publications.

Dr. Shankland sees patients from all over North, South and Central America, Europe, Africa, Asia, and the Caribbean. He welcomes new patients.

In his spare time, Dr. Shankland is president of three Internet companies. He enjoys writing short stories, three of which have been published to date. He's currently working on a book of short stories. Dr. Shankland is also a martial artist (Shorin-ryu karate [Okinawan karate-do] and Hung Gar fung fu).

Index

A

E

Eagle's Syndrome 108, 114-116
Earache 59, 61, 68
Ears 123, 179, 207, 224, 225, 227
Elavil 174, 175
Endocarditis 74, 84
Endodontic Therapy 81
Endoscopy 133
Ernest, Dr. Edwin 7, 109, 112
Ernest Syndrome 108, 112-116, 234
Essential Oils 209, 213-217
Esters 215
Ethnic Differences 29
Eucalyptus 217

F

Face 13, 127, 129, 225
Facial Nerve 113, 126-128
Factitious Disorders 23
Family Influences 28
Feverfew 210
Fibromyalgia 141-146, 151, 195
Flexeril 187
Focal Theory of Infection 81, 82, 85
Foramen, Apical 57
Fothergill, John 46
Frey's Neuralgia 108, 125

G

Gamma Knife 50
Gasserian Ganglion 50, 120
Gastric Reflux 89
Gattefosse, Rene 214
Geranium 215, 217
Ginger 210
Gingiva 74, 78
Gingivitis 73-76, 79
Glossodynia 88, 89
Glossopharyngeal Neuralgia 108, 122, 123

Glucose intolerance 89
Glycerin 47, 49
Glycerol 47, 52
Goldenseal 210
Grape 79
Grinding 163
Guiafenesin 152
Guilt 28, 31-33, 39

H

Hahnemann, Dr. Samuel 193
Hamular Process 108, 117-120
Hayes, Woody 64
Head 16, 46, 50, 69, 124, 138, 140, 221, 223, 225
Headache 16, 31, 109, 115, 133, 139, 140, 161, 162, 166, 196, 201, 225
Heparin 102
Herbal Medicine 209
Herpes Simplex 127, 150
Herpes Zoster 123, 124, 210
Histamine 145, 146
Homeopathic 71, 84, 192, 194
Homeopathy 102, 191-196
Horehound 210
Hormonal Changes 90
Hormones 146, 147, 169, 204
HPA Axis 146, 147, 152
Hunter, William 81
Hygienist 58, 65, 74, 77
Hyperbaric 103

I

Ibuprofen 61, 67, 176, 180-184
Implants 82, 97
Infarction 74, 84, 95, 96, 100
Infective Endocarditis 74, 84
Informational Substances 144
Ionic Channels 212
Ischemia 95, 96
Ischemic Heart Disease 83
Ischemic Osteonecrosis 94, 97, 100

O

P

R